Boost your Energy

Dr Sandra Cabot M.B.B.S., D.R.C.O.G., is a well-known media doctor and author of the best-selling books: *Women's Health, Don't Let Your Hormones Ruin Your Life, The Body-Shaping Diet, Menopause—HRT and Its Natural Alternatives, Handbag Health Guide* and *The Liver-Cleansing Diet*.

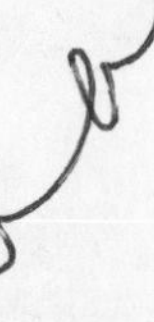

Sandra is a consultant to the Australian Women's Health Advisory Service, has regularly appeared in many Australian TV shows, has her own talk-back radio show, writes for women's magazines and is a much sought after public speaker on women's health, hormonal disorders and naturopathic medicine.

Sandra is sometimes known as the 'flying doctor' as she frequently flies herself to many of Australia's country towns to hold health forums for rural women. These help to raise funds for local women's health services. She spent considerable time working in the Department of Obstetrics and Gynaecology in a large missionary hospital in the Himalayan foothills of India.

Sandra has communicated with women via TV and radio and receives thousands of letters from women all over the world. Thus she is acutely aware of the health problems and needs of women from many different backgrounds.

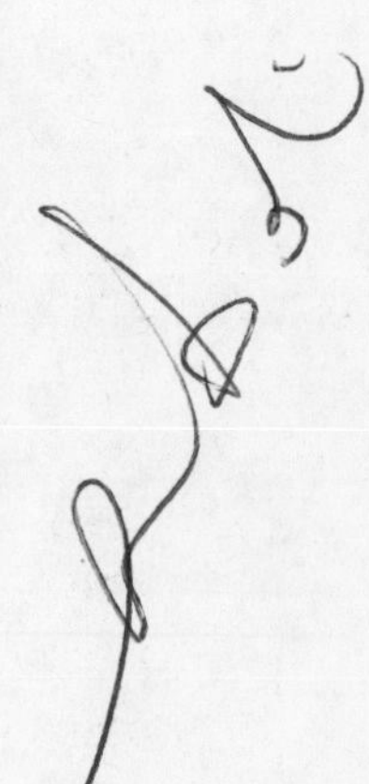

Boost your Energy

Dr Sandra Cabot

Womens' Health Advisory Service

email: cabot@ozemail.com.au

Internet: www.whas.com.au

The suggestions, ideas and treatments described in this book are not intended to replace the care and supervision of a trained health professional. All problems and concerns regarding your health require medical supervision. If you have any pre-existing medical disorders you must consult your doctor before following any suggestions or treatments in this book. If you are taking prescription medications you should check with your own doctor before using any of the treatments discussed in this book.

First published 1997 by
WHAS
PO Box 217, Paddington, NSW, 2021, Australia
email: cabot@ozemail.com.au
Internet: www.whas.com.au
Edited by Carolyn Child
Designed by Karen Stirling and Murray Child of Murray David Publishing Pty Ltd

ISBN 0 646339 46 X

Our delightful cartoons were drawn by
the talented artist Karen Barbouttis

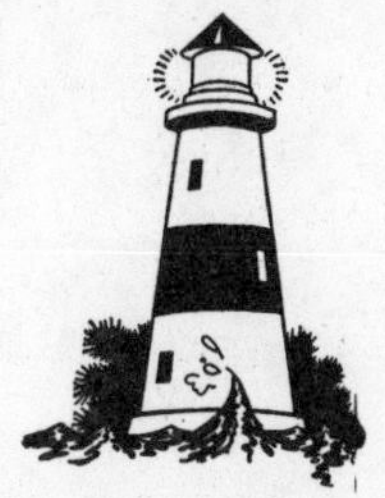

This book is dedicated to under-privileged women and homeless teenagers.

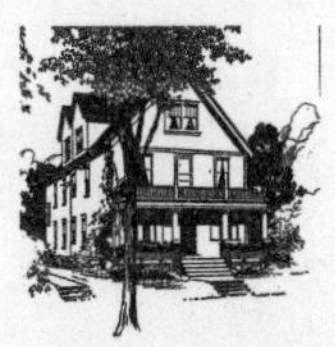

For every book sold, a donation is given to Samaritan House women's refuge in New South Wales and The Lighthouse Foundation for homeless teenagers in Victoria.

Thank you for your support!

Contents

TESTIMONIALS

A POLICEMAN FROM SYDNEY

Dear Dr Cabot,

After working irregular hours as a shift worker, I started to feel constantly tired both mentally and physically. After seeing numerous doctors, naturopaths and other alternative health practitioners, all of whom were unable to help, I resigned myself to the fact that it was just a result of modern-day living. One thing the naturopaths agreed upon was that my liver was not functioning properly. So I purchased a liver tonic powder and also the ingredients mentioned in your 'energy cocktail'.

As I work irregular hours, I have not been able to properly follow all of your dietary recommendations. I have, however, made a point of taking the liver tonic and your energy cocktail on a daily basis.

I am happy to say that my energy level has increased significantly and I am now motivated enough to resume exercise, which in turn increases my level of energy and feeling of well-being. Your energy cocktail alone is well worth the price of your book and, when time permits, I look forward to starting your diet.

MRS J. K. FROM PERTH

Dear Dr Cabot,

I am writing to let you know that I have finally regained my energy using your technique of fine-tuning the body and it is such a great relief. I am only 45, yet six months ago I felt 85 and had to give up my job because I could not meet my commitments. My fatigue started three weeks after having a hysterectomy, during which my ovaries and uterus were removed because of severe endometriosis. I thought that I was strong enough to recover with a good diet alone and I also began taking some oestrogen tablets because I started an instant menopause. Unfortunately, I started to develop aches and pains, headaches, nausea and chronic fatigue. I had no libido and indeed I could not stand my husband to touch me, which caused a lot of stress as his energy levels were high. Then I read an article of yours on the subject of fine-tuning the body with natural hormones and nutritional supplements. This struck a chord with me as I knew that my body needed more help and that it must be lacking something, as I felt way out of balance. I had some blood tests done to measure my hormones and I found that I had very low levels of testosterone and DHEA, although my oestrogen levels were high. I discussed this with my doctor who prescribed some hormone lozenges containing small amounts of the hormones testosterone and pregnenolone and changed me to the oestrogen patches. I took your advice and started taking some nutritional supplements containing magnesium, selenium, vitamin C and essential fatty acids. I also started having one of your energy shakes containing LSA and raw juices everyday. Within six weeks I could start to feel my body responding and I felt stronger and more alive mentally and sexually. It was as if my body was receiving the substances that it needed to rebalance and restore its energy production. I am now feeling superb and I cannot believe that I feel like this everyday. My family are so pleased to have found the mother and wife and indeed the happy human being that they used to know.

MRS T. S. FROM ADELAIDE

Dear Dr Cabot,

I have been a chronic fatigue syndrome sufferer for three years and found that I always had sore throats and swollen glands. I had a lot of mucous build up in my sinuses and was always taking different antibiotics which gave me candida. Luckily, I then came across your liver-cleansing diet and it really made sense to me because I knew that my immune system needed help. I followed this diet for eight weeks and the sore throats and mucous gradually went; however, I still felt worn out and lack lustre. So I decided that my immune system needed building up and I decided to take the supplements you recommend for boosting energy. I went to the health food store and purchased anti-oxidants, a designer yeast powder to give me selenium and trace minerals, flaxseed oil and some capsules containing the three herbs guarana, ginkgo and ginseng. I also started on some magnesium tablets because I had a high stress job. Well, after five weeks I began to feel my energy levels increasing and I no longer felt sleepy in the afternoons. Even better, I felt great when I awakened in the mornings and did not crave sugar and coffee to get me going. I can truly say that nutritional therapy has cured my problems and I hate to think what my future would have been if I had not discovered it.

TESTIMONIALS

MR P. D. FROM TAREE, NSW

Dear Dr Sandra Cabot,

I am writing to tell you of my success after changing my diet and lifestyle. I am 48 years old and I have had high blood pressure for five years which necessitated the use of a beta blocker drug to slow my heart and keep the blood pressure from soaring. Unfortunately, the beta blockers made me feel very tired and I was not able to perform sexually which gave me low self-esteem. After reading your Liver-Cleansing Diet *book I decided that I really wanted to change so I stopped eating the unhealthy fats and salty foods and started eating a lot of raw food. I read something you had written about magnesium and coenzyme Q10 to help the circulation, so I started taking magnesium 2000 mg daily and coenzyme Q10 100 mg daily. I also started to relax more and walk every day which helped to relieve my cold hands and feet. I have lost 15 kilograms in weight and my bowels have become regular for the first time in years. My doctor is very pleased with my blood pressure and now the only medication that I need to take is a diuretic tablet which is not very strong. The magnesium seems to control my blood pressure and racing heart, but the best thing of all for me is that I can now have a normal sex life which has made me feel like the man I used to be. Thank you very much for my new lease of life.*

HERE IS AN EMAIL FROM MRS J. S., CYBERSPACE, SOMEWHERE IN AUSTRALIA

Dear Dr Cabot,

I just wanted to email you and let you know that I have been on the Liver-Cleansing Diet for five weeks now and feel great. I use to suffer from regular headaches (at least one every two days), and at least once a week get a migraine which would knock me out for 12 to 15 hours at a time. Since I started the diet, I feel great, have lost 6 kilos and haven't been in a bad mood since this time. My neighbour got me onto it and I have told everyone I know about it. Now people are always commenting on how great I look and want to know why (they think I must have a new man in my life). I keep telling them that it is your book. Basically, I just wanted to thank you for myself and my daughter, who no longer has this 'bitch from hell mother' four days a week. I am only 25 but it is the best thing I have ever come across and I have been on and off diets since I was 18. Keep up the good work!!

CHAPTER ONE

INCREASE YOUR ENERGY

As a doctor I see hundreds of patients who complain of lack of energy. They have lost their 'oomph' or *joie de vivre* and many have been like this for years. They may complain of fatigue in the mornings which makes it hard to face the challenges of a new day or they may be just plain tired all the time. Often there will be a lack of physical and mental energy and it is difficult to know which comes first as both will exacerbate each other.

In this book we will give you strategies for:

1. MENTAL FATIGUE
2. HORMONAL FATIGUE
3. NUTRITIONAL FATIGUE
4. CHRONIC FATIGUE SYNDROME

There are solutions for chronic fatigue because, thankfully, in this day and age we are able to **fine-tune the body and mind** to rejuvenate our hormonal system, immune system, muscular system and nervous system.

I will give you the **tools** to do this so that your body, which is like a finely-tuned instrument, can be invigorated and balanced. I love the subject of fine-tuning because after more than twenty years in medicine I have discovered that everyone is an individual and only with the tools of nutritional and hormonal medicine, tailor-made for every person, can we restore the balance of energy. These tools enable us to fine-tune every cell of our body so that the biochemical pathways and energy factories inside the cells are stimulated to produce optimum energy. We are all made up of billions of cells and to achieve optimum health every cell must be given the raw materials for maximum energy output. We are working on the microscopic world of the cell and changing the tiny molecules within it.

The idea of **'fine-tuning'** the body is very new as it is only in this day and age that it has become possible. We could also use the term **'ultra-tuning'** the body to produce ultimate energy. Mechanics will relate to the term 'ultra-tuning' as they know the huge difference in the performance of an engine that this form of maintenance can achieve. To me it is a sad oversight that we will spend the time and money to ultra-tune our car engines and yet no-one bothers to perform this vital maintenance upon their own body. Our own body is the ultimate engine and needs the best fuel and fine-tuning to give maximum performance if it is to run efficiently and have a long life.

We need to fine-tune or ultra-tune our bodies regularly to prevent deterioration and not wait until symptoms of dysfunction or disease supervene. Fine-tuning is not only vital for the effective cure of diseases, it is also the ultimate form of preventative medicine.

Every cell in your body has the genetic code (DNA) which programs it to function perfectly; however, if your cells do not have the right raw materials to carry out the genetic messages given to the cell, imbalances will result. Fine-tuning provides your cells with these vital raw materials to allow the cellular genetic code to express itself fully. This is as close to perfect health as you can ever get.

Fine-tuning or ultra-tuning the body and mind is an exciting journey which will profoundly change the way you look and feel physically and mentally.

THE PRODUCTION OF ENERGY

Before we get into the nitty-gritty of how to overcome the various causes of fatigue, I thought it may be interesting to describe how our cells actually make the energy required to sustain the function of our organs. If you do not like physiology please feel free to skip this small section because it is only included for interest.

The energy factories of our cells are the **mitochondria** (see page 9) which are tiny bean-shaped structures made of layers of fatty membranes. By a chemical process called the **Krebs cycle,** food is turned into the currency of cellular energy, which is a chemical called Adenosine Triphosphate (ATP). The Krebs cycle occurs inside the little mitochondria and requires oxygen (aerobic metabolism) and this is coupled to an electron chain transport system. The more ATP that is produced, the more energy the cell will have, that is why we call ATP the currency of energy. This Krebs cycle accounts for approximately 75 per cent of the total energy produced in the cell. From page 8, you can see that fats, carbohydrates and proteins are converted most efficiently into energy via the Krebs cycle in the mitochondria. You can see also that various nutritional co-factors are required in the Krebs cycle such as lipoic acid, various B vitamins, L-carnitine, magnesium, manganese, amino acids, maleic acid and coenzyme Q10.

L-carnitine (see Krebs cycle) is the shovel that puts fuel into the mitochondria and is essential for energy production. L-carnitine is made in the body from the essential amino acids lysine and methionine and also requires the co-factors vitamins B_3, B_6, C and iron for

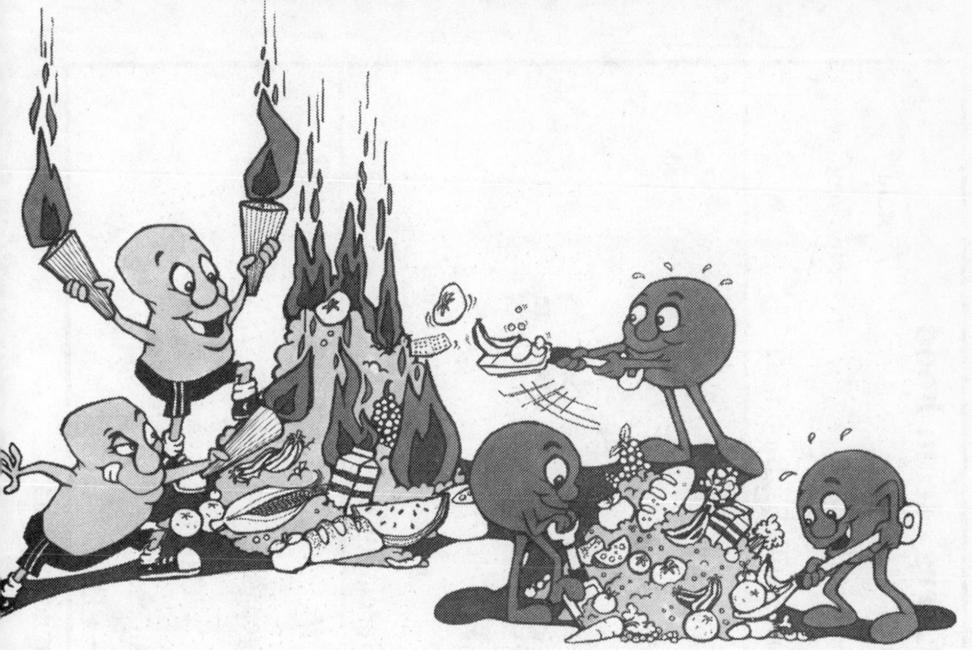

L-carnitine shovels food into the energy factory, to enhance energy production from the mitochondria, which work to burn fuel to ensure the body's production of energy will be adequate.

its production. These co-factors can be obtained from the energy diet and also through specific nutritional supplements if required.

The cell also has another way of producing energy in its inner liquid (cytoplasm) which does not require oxygen (anaerobic metabolism). In anaerobic metabolism the cell converts sugar (glucose) into lactate; however, this is not very efficient and accounts for a much smaller amount of cellular energy than does the aerobic Krebs cycle.

If the mitochondria are not working properly the cell may be forced to rely too much on anaerobic metabolism in the cytoplasm and a build up of acidic waste products may then occur, leading to muscular aches and pains, cravings for sugar and fatigue. Thus, we need to ensure that our mitochondria are working efficiently by providing them with all the essential raw materials they require for an

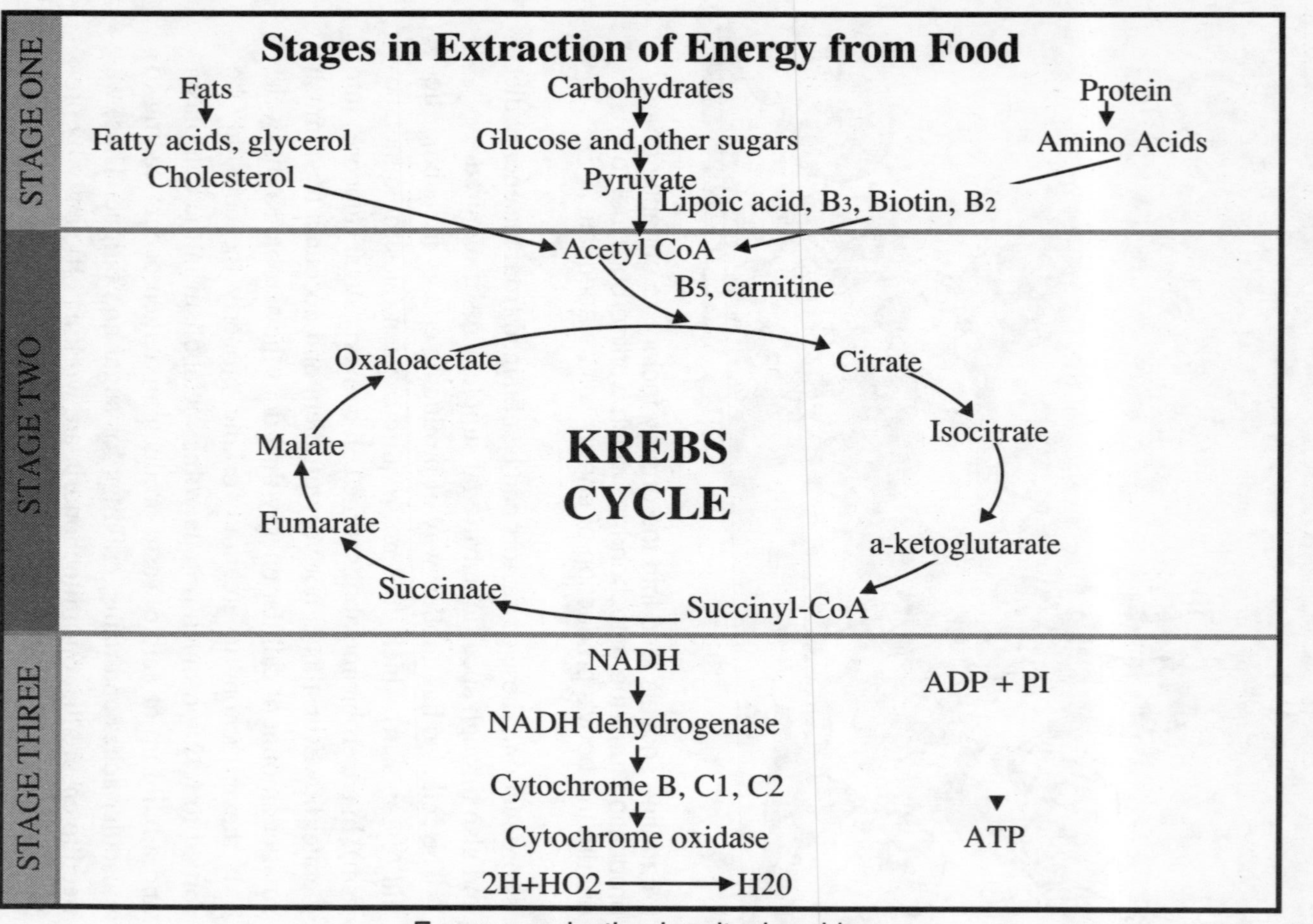

Energy production in mitochondria.

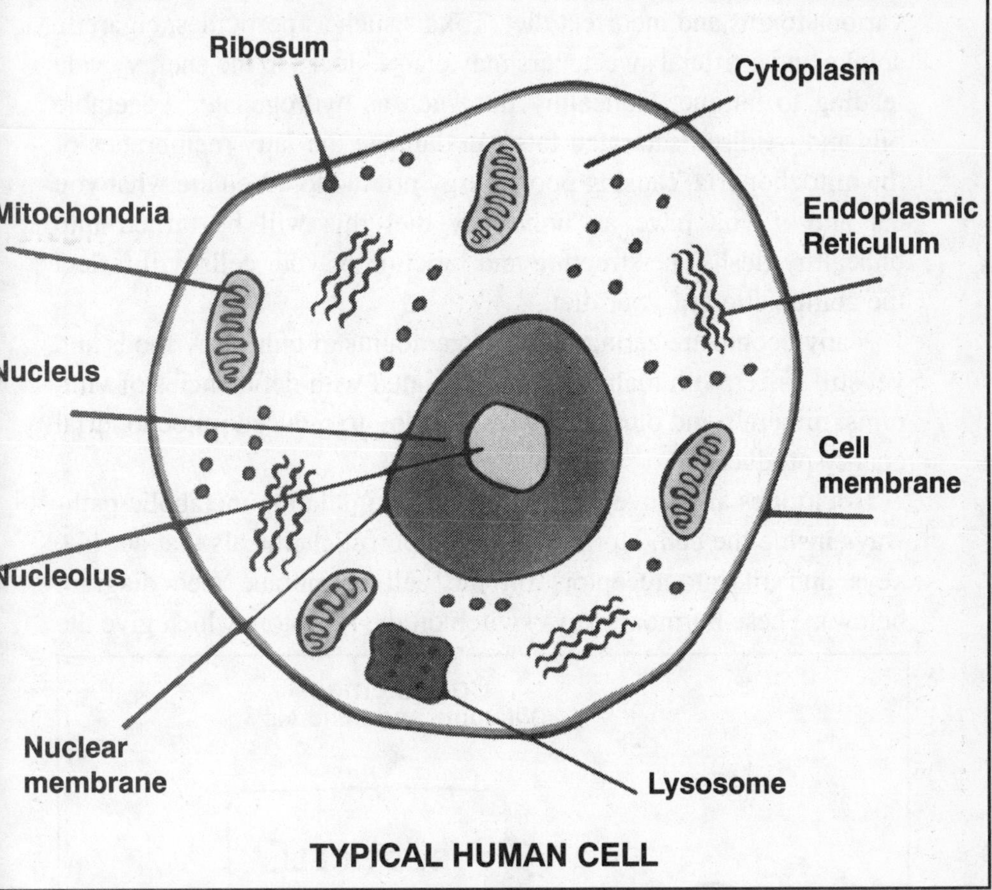

TYPICAL HUMAN CELL

efficient Krebs cycle. The energy diet and the nutrients in my fine-tuning cocktail (see page 202) will provide the mitochondria with adequate raw materials (substrates) for an efficient Krebs cycle and thus for efficient energy production. The mitochondria are made up of fatty membranes and may be damaged by viruses, toxins and free radicals.

Anti-oxidants (such as vitamins A, C, E, and selenium) and essential fatty acids will reduce damage to the mitochondria, thus helping to preserve energy.

The energy cycle within the mitochondria can be blocked by

various toxins and incorrect diet. Toxins such as pesticides, cigarette smoke and artificial sweeteners may cause blocks in the energy cycle leading to fatigue. Unhealthy fats such as hydrogenated vegetable oils and oxidised saturated fats can damage the fatty membranes of the mitochondria, causing poor energy production. You are what you eat and if you have an unhealthy diet this will be turned into unhealthy flesh. The structure and function of your cells will reflect the composition of your diet.

Many people are eating excessive amounts of unhealthy foods and yet still suffer with malnutrition associated with deficiencies of vitamins, minerals and other nutrients, leading to reduced mitochondrial energy production.

Hormones also have a role to play in stimulating metabolic pathways inside the cell. Hormones are powerful chemicals that act like keys and fit into receptors on the cell membrane (see diagram below). These hormonal keys switch on the receptors which give the

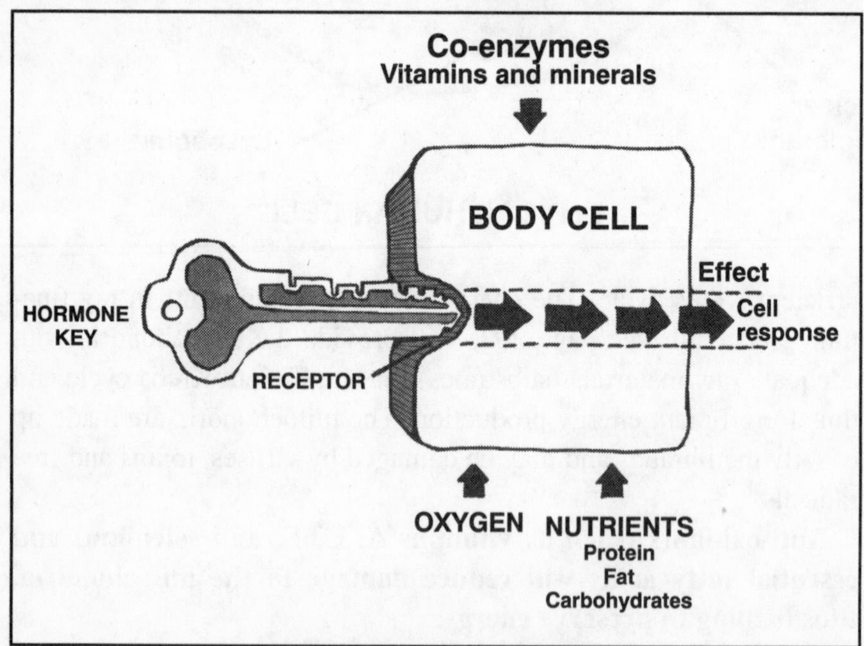

THE HEALTHY CELL

cell various messages—for example, to make more proteins or secretions. So hormones are like managers and give your cells directions to follow. Some hormones, such as sex steroids and some adrenal hormones, cause your cells to act like younger cells and enable you to function like a younger person. Because of the ageing population it is important for us to know that the production of some significant hormones unfortunately diminishes with age. In this book we consider the use of the most important anti-ageing hormones which can rejuvenate the cells.

To achieve optimal health the tiny molecules and microscopic components of every cell in the body must be in balance and working efficiently. The technique of fine-tuning works on this microscopic level and incorporates the balancing of hormones and vital nutrients to create and maintain cellular efficiency and peak physiological function. It also considers cellular protection and the immune system because we live in a world where the environment has become more hostile to the cells and with advancing age our cells also become more prone to damage and inefficiency.

Fine-tuning is truly a total and comprehensive technique for health restoration and maintenance because it considers all the vital factors required for cellular performance and longevity.

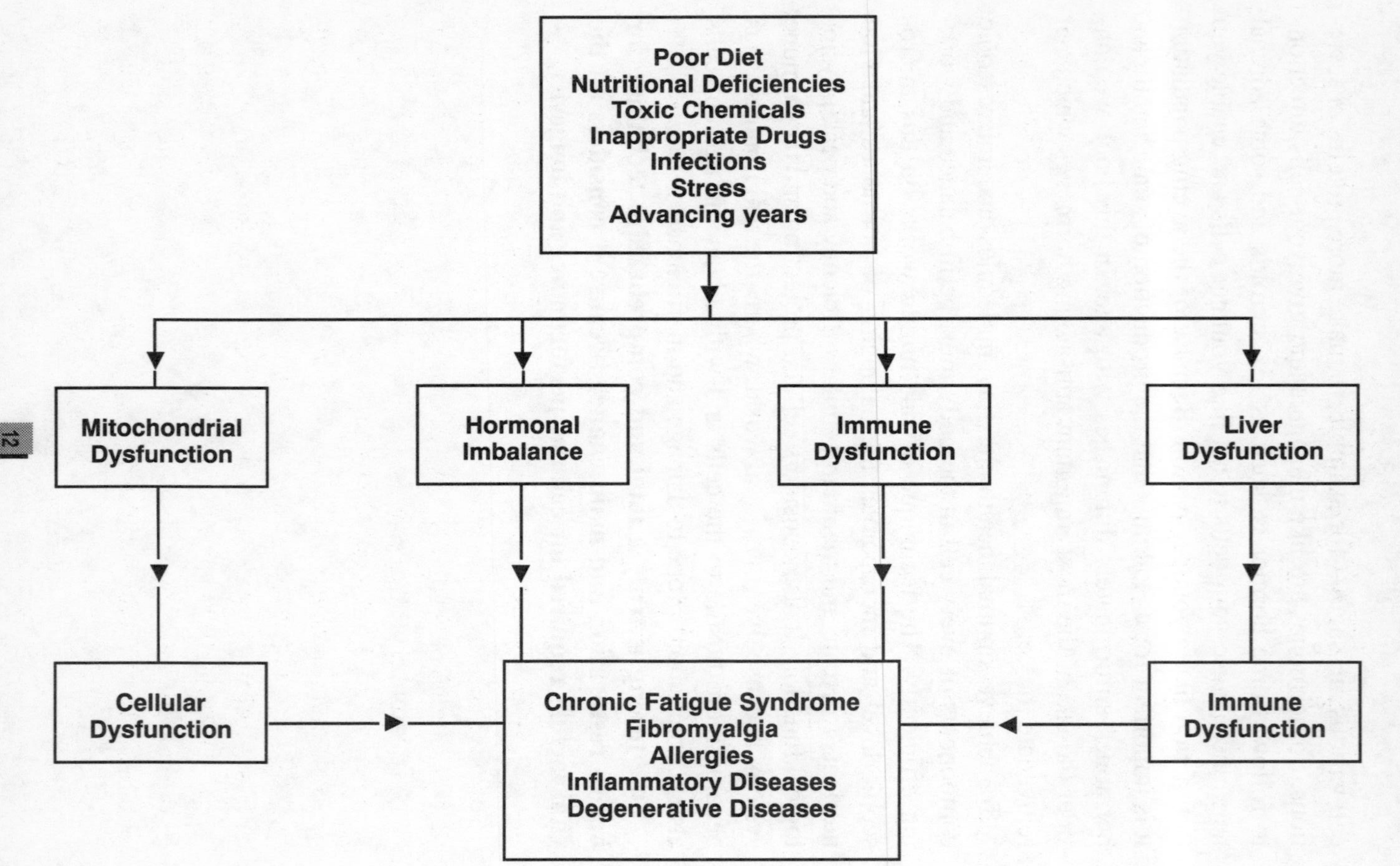
Poor Diet
Nutritional Deficiencies
Toxic Chemicals
Inappropriate Drugs
Infections
Stress
Advancing years
Mitochondrial Dysfunction
Hormonal Imbalance
Immune Dysfunction
Liver Dysfunction
Cellular Dysfunction
Chronic Fatigue Syndrome
Fibromyalgia
Allergies
Inflammatory Diseases
Degenerative Diseases
Immune Dysfunction

CHAPTER TWO

BOOSTING MENTAL ENERGY

If the production of energy in the brain is suboptimal you may suffer from depression, lack of concentration, 'foggy' brain, loss of mental drive, sleep disturbances, poor memory, lack of interest and mood disorders.

If these symptoms are severe and stop you from functioning, you may need to consult a specialist psychiatrist who will give you counselling and perhaps anti-depressant drugs. I am not against these things and indeed they may be extremely beneficial. However, you will probably want to come off these drugs sooner or later and you will surely want to know of more natural solutions to stop these unpleasant symptoms recurring. Here are my suggestions to balance the production of neurochemicals (neurotransmitters) in the brain cells.

SUPPLEMENTS TO BOOST MENTAL ENERGY AND PRODUCTIVITY

1. **Lecithin,** 4000 mg daily, will give extra choline to increase levels of the brain transmitter acetylcholine. To increase the effect of choline take the lecithin with vitamin B_5 (pantothenic acid), 500 mg daily, vitamin B_6 (pyridoxine), 100 mg daily and vitamin B_1 (thiamine), 100 mg daily. Take all the above with food. These nutrients will help improve your memory. You should also eat foods high in choline, such as soya beans, split peas, lentils, green beans, eggs, lean beef and bean sprouts.
2. **Essential fatty acids,** such as evening primrose oil, 3000–4000 mg daily and flaxseed oil (also known as linseed), 3000–4000 mg daily, will provide your brain with a good balance of omega 6 and omega 3 fatty acids which will help the brain cells in many ways.

Essential fatty acids are the building blocks of the fatty membranes that form the structural integrity of your brain cells. The brain is a soft fatty organ, largely composed of fats called phospholipids.

By taking essential fatty acids you will improve the release of neurotransmitters from your brain cells, thereby increasing your mental acuity. As the population ages the incidence of dementia, especially Alzheimer's disease, is increasing at an alarming rate. The genesis of dementia is related to loss of brain cells causing atrophy (shrinkage) of the brain. These brain cells shrink and die because they have weak leaky membranes which are incapable of protecting the cells. Their mitochondria, which are also made of fatty membranes, are inefficient, causing amyloid tissue (metabolic garbage) to build up within the brain cells, eventually choking them to death. To reduce your chances of dementia it is imperative that you supply your brain cells with adequate essential fatty acids to build strong healthy membranes on the inside and outside of the cells.

ALZHEIMER'S DISEASE

This is a common form of dementia which causes loss of short-term memory and the ability to think logically. Unfortunately, this tragic degenerative brain disease affects around 10 per cent of people over sixty-five years of age.

In Alzheimer's patients we see characteristic physical changes in the brain consisting of deposits of a useless protein called beta-amyloid. These deposits take the shape of plaques and a tangled web and literally start to take over the brain, killing precious brain cells in their path.

Researchers have found that flawed genes, such as APP and Presenilin I, can act like a throttle and accelerate the formation of the beta-amyloid deposits in the brain. They can also reduce cell repair and accelerate cell death in the brain.

Researcher, David Borchett of Johns Hopkins Medical Institute in Baltimore, inserted these two flawed genes into mice, one at a time. When the APP flawed gene was inserted alone, amyloid plaques developed late in the life span of the mice. When both flawed genes were inserted, these plaques developed at a much earlier stage. Thus, the flawed gene Presenilin I speeds up the onset of Alzheimer's disease (AD).

Poor diet and nutritional deficiencies can accelerate the onset of AD, both directly by their effect upon brain cells (neurones) and indirectly by interacting with flawed genes. Deficiencies of dietary essential fatty acids will lead to poor quality cell membranes in the brain cells, which are more susceptible to free radical damage.

Nutritional deficiencies can cause poor energy production in the mitochondria which deprives the brain cells of the energy required to prevent and remove build up of amyloid deposits within them. Deficiencies of the B vitamins B1, B3, B12 and folic acid and the minerals zinc and magnesium can reduce mitochondrial energy production and these deficiencies have been found to be more common in people who develop AD. Reference 30, Henry Osieki, *Physicians Handbook of Clinical Nutrition*, Bioconcepts Publishing.

Cells starved of their own internal supply of energy because of poor mitochondrial function do not have the energy reserves to prevent or remove amyloid deposits, So the amyloid continues to build up inside the cells and gradually chokes the cells to death. A deficiency of anti-oxidants can increase the susceptibility of the brain cell membranes to free radical damage.

An important anti-oxidant for the prevention of AD is vitamin E. A recent study in the *New England Journal of Medicine* (Reference 35) found that the progression of AD is slowed with

1000 IU of vitamin E twice daily. I recommend that not only vitamin E, but the full spectrum of important anti-oxidants—namely vitamin C, selenium and beta-carotene—must be obtained from the diet and supplements to give a comprehensive shield against free radical damage to neurones.

Avoid eating large or regular amounts of damaged fats such as rancid (oxidised) fats found in deep fried foods and preserved meats or trans-fatty acids found in margarine or hydrogenated vegetable oils. These fats have a deleterious effect upon cell membranes, including those of neurones.

Toxic chemicals which can act as cellular poisons in the brain can increase the risk of dementia. Pesticides and insecticides are fat-soluble chemicals which are readily stored in the fatty parts of the brain. They act as mitochondrial poisons, reducing cellular energy production and also block the function of the brain chemical called acetyl-choline which is a neurotransmitter involved with memory. If the liver is overloaded and cannot break down these toxins, much larger amounts find their way into the brain. Thus, poor liver function can be a risk factor for toxin-induced brain damage. Other potential mitochondrial toxins that may impair memory are lead, aluminium, mercury and fluoride and can be reduced by using a good quality water filter.

Supplements to improve memory and reduce the risk of Alzheimer's disease

1. Vitamin E, 1000 IU, twice daily.
2. Vitamin C, 1000 mg, daily.
3. Selenium, 100 mcg, daily.
4. Vitamin B complex, one tablet every second day.
5. Essential fatty acids from supplements and the diet (see page 71).

6. Lipoic acid, 100 mg daily. This is an anti-oxidant that neutralises dangerous peroxynitrite free radicals.
7. Acetyl-carnitine, 200 mg three times daily. This is able to boost mitochondrial energy and increase production of the memory neurotransmitter acetylcholine.
8. Phosphatidyl-serine, 100 mg three times daily to increase production of acetyl-choline.

References 36 and 37.

Nutritional medicine can help to prevent and treat AD. It is most successful if it is begun early in the disease when a big improvement in mental function is often achieved. Even in those with flawed genes, nutritional medicine can greatly delay or prevent the onset of degenerative diseases such as AD. Nutritional medicine can repair some types of flawed genes, can prevent these genes from expressing themselves fully and can repair the metabolic damage that they cause. Those with a family history of AD would be wise to use diet and nutritional supplements from the time of adulthood to reduce their risk.

3. **Amino acids** are the building blocks of the neurotransmitters and those with a strict vegetarian diet or digestive problems may have deficiencies of some of the essential amino acids. This can lead to mental fatigue and mood disorders. If you are a strict vegetarian or have a poor appetite I recommend that you take both an amino acid supplement and **spirulina** at least twice daily.

   If your diet contains animal products and yet you still have mental fatigue and feel moody, you may find that supplements of **single specific amino acids** can be extremely helpful. This should be supervised by a naturopath or a doctor with an interest in nutritional medicine. Amino acids in high doses are generally safe; however, they should not be taken with anti-depressant drugs.

If you feel sluggish and depressed and want to sit in a chair and do nothing all day, you may find that supplements of the single amino acids **tyrosine** and **phenylalanine** will restore your well-being. Tyrosine and phenylalanine will increase the levels of the brain chemicals norepinephrine and dopamine which have a **stimulant** action.

If you feel very moody and uptight, with poor sleep and lack of sex drive and you do not enjoy things anymore, you can increase your levels of the brain chemical called serotonin by taking the single amino acid **tryptophan.**

If your thought processes are too slow and you are not as 'switched on' as you used to be, you may find that a supplement of the single amino acid L-glutamine will give you the extra mental acuity (similar to the RAM memory in a computer) that you require. **L-glutamine** will increase the levels of glutamine and the important regulating neurotransmitter GABA in the brain. It has also been found to help reduce the craving for alcohol.

All single amino supplements should be taken only with carbohydrates or a sweet drink because if they are taken with protein foods they will not pass through the blood-brain barrier efficiently.

4. **Melatonin** is a natural hormone produced from the pineal gland at the base of the brain. It is secreted as our eyes register the fall of darkness and promotes a sound restful sleep. During 1995 melatonin became the biggest health craze ever to hit America and health food stores could not keep it on the shelf. The craze was fuelled by best-selling books such as *The Melatonin Miracle* by Drs Walter Pierpaoli and William Regelson and *Melatonin: Nature's Sleeping Pill* by Dr Ray Sahelian. Low-dose supplements of the hormone melatonin can hasten sleep, overcome jet lag without the side effects of prescription sleeping pills and can help to slow down the ageing process. Hordes of Americans are finding the lure of a natural and cheap panacea

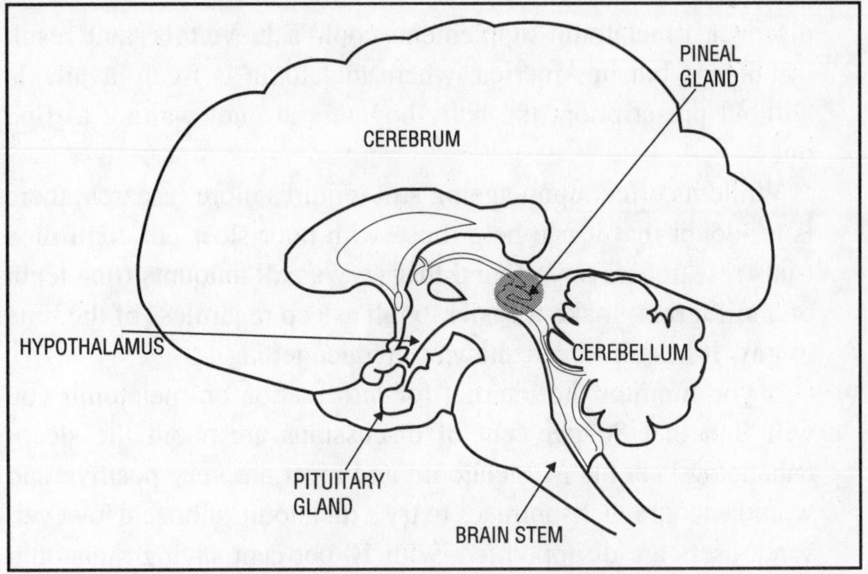

The pineal gland produces melatonin.

simply irresistible, so much so that melatonin has created a health revolution.

This craze has been good for the health food stores and publishers but should millions of consumers be taking melatonin like jelly beans? Melatonin may slow the biological clock within us; however, no-one has ever studied the long-term effects of using melatonin in humans. Humans, like animals, produce large amounts of melatonin early in life, with blood levels dropping sharply at puberty, then melatonin production continues to decline gradually as we age. Dr Pierpaoli wondered if this decline had anything to do with ageing and set about to prove this by surgically switching the pineal glands of ten young mice with ten old mice. This gave the old mice youthful levels of melatonin at the youngsters' expense. The outcome was fascinating as the young mice with the old pineal glands became weak and died in late middle age, whereas the old mice extended their life expectancies by around 30 per cent! It would take twenty to thirty years to discover if melatonin supplements could achieve this same result in humans but in America, where melatonin is freely available without prescription, the baby boomers are not waiting to find out.

While its effect upon ageing still requires more research, there is no doubt that it can help those with poor sleep. In controlled trials researchers have found that very small amounts (one tenth of a milligram) make it easier to fall asleep regardless of the time of day. It has also been shown to reduce jet lag.

If you monitor the internet for information on melatonin you will find that 80 per cent of discussions are about the sleep-enhancing benefits of melatonin and most are very positive and would encourage insomniacs to try a melatonin snooze. However, some users are disappointed, with 10 per cent saying melatonin did not work at all and 10 per cent complaining of side effects, such as bad dreams, headaches, morning grogginess, mild depression and poor libido. Despite the surge in melatonin use the American Food and Drug Administration (FDA) has not received many complaints about side effects. Reported side effects were disrupted sleep, genital pain and nausea and the FDA could not be sure they were due to melatonin as the complaints were so small in number. However, some health experts sound a word of caution and believe that too many people are playing with a potent hormone before the jury is back in. One must question the high doses some people are taking, as even one milligram is three times higher than the normal amount produced by the pineal gland. High doses could have unknown long-term effects. Another worry is that in the USA there is no regulation of the quality or quantity of melatonin sold in the shops because the FDA does not monitor the sale of dietary supplements. Melatonin is sold in America as a dietary supplement which seems strange considering that it is a hormone!

In Australia, melatonin is available on prescription and if you would like more information contact compounding pharmacist Mr Richard Stenlake at 169 Oxford Street, Bondi Junction, NSW, 2022. Melatonin is safer than sleeping pills and is not addictive; however, there are some people who should avoid it for now, at least until more is known about its risks. These are: pregnant or nursing mothers, people with auto-immune diseases, severe allergies, or cancers of the immune system (such as lymphoma or leukaemia) and normal children who already produce high levels. It is also wise to avoid it if you are trying to conceive because high doses of melatonin act as a contraceptive.

Currently, melatonin is a potentially useful hormone that the health food industry in America is rushing to sell. I would feel more comfortable if it was kept in the medical arena and made available only on a doctor's prescription. Interestingly, the pineal gland increases production of melatonin after some forms of meditation which is why people who practise this ancient technique feel so calm and content.

The loss of melatonin is thought to be one of the reasons why, as we age, sleep disturbances, fatigue and anxiety are more common. If you find yourself in this situation I believe it is worthwhile trying a supplement of the hormone melatonin because in a significant percentage of people it works very well and definitely does not cause the side effects of sleeping tablets or sedatives. It should be prescribed by a doctor and is usually taken in a dose of 1–3 mg around the time of sunset. For more information you could read the book *Stay Young the Melatonin Way,* published by Random House.

CHAPTER THREE

OVERCOMING HORMONAL FATIGUE

Imbalances in the production of hormones can lead to sluggish metabolism and fluctuating energy levels. The most common imbalances occur in the production of hormones from the thyroid gland, the sex glands and the adrenal glands and quite often they may occur simultaneously.

THYROID IMBALANCES

The thyroid gland, situated in front of your neck (over the Adam's apple), produces thyroid hormone in the form of thyroxine (let's call it T4) and pumps it out into the bloodstream. This T4 is taken in by your cells where it is converted to the **active form** of thyroid hormone called triidothyronine (let's call it T3). T3 has a stimulating effect upon the cells which increases the metabolic rate, so helping your cells to utilise food energy more efficiently. This process must occur continually if you are to keep your energy levels up and your weight under control. There are several steps in this process where things can go wrong. For example, the thyroid gland may not produce enough T4 hormone and this condition is called **hypothyroidism** which means an underactive thyroid gland. This problem can be overcome by taking thyroxine (T4) tablets every day along with a selection of supplements, such as kelp, magnesium, vitamin E, selenium and flaxseed oil capsules.

Another problem that can occur is inefficient conversion of the T4 hormone to the active form of thyroid hormone T3. This is known as thyroid resistance. If you have **thyroid resistance** you will probably need to take two forms of thyroid hormone tablets (both T4 and T3) in order to restore the balance of energy in your cells. T4 tablets are

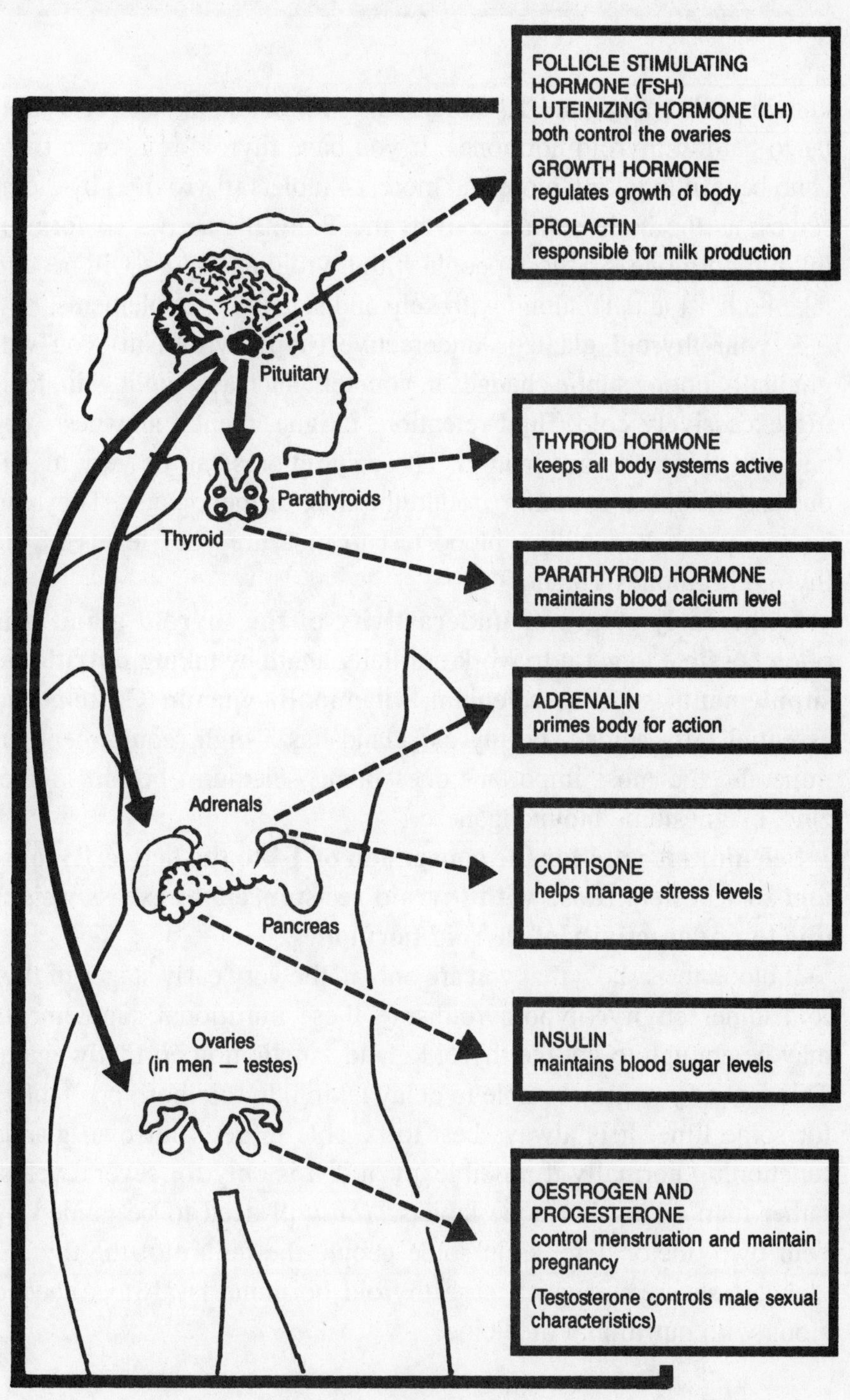
FOLLICLE STIMULATING HORMONE (FSH)
LUTEINIZING HORMONE (LH)
both control the ovaries
GROWTH HORMONE
regulates growth of body
PROLACTIN
responsible for milk production
Pituitary
THYROID HORMONE
keeps all body systems active
Parathyroids
Thyroid
PARATHYROID HORMONE
maintains blood calcium level
ADRENALIN
primes body for action
Adrenals
CORTISONE
helps manage stress levels
Pancreas
INSULIN
maintains blood sugar levels
Ovaries
(in men — testes)
OESTROGEN AND PROGESTERONE
control menstruation and maintain pregnancy
(Testosterone controls male sexual characteristics)

known as thyroxine and T3 tablets as tertroxin and have effects similar to natural thyroid hormones. If you have thyroid resistance there is no benefit in taking more and more T4 tablets (thyroxine) by themselves, as the body cannot convert the T4 to the active T3 form of thyroid hormone. So those people with thyroid resistance will need to take both T4 and T3 along with kelp and selenium supplements.

If your thyroid gland is underactive (hypothyroidism) you will gradually notice subtle changes in yourself, such as weight gain, feeling excessively cold, fluid retention, fatigue, mental slowness, dry hair and skin and constipation. These symptoms can be very insidious and are more common around the time of menopause. They can be easily checked with a blood test to measure your levels of the thyroid hormones T3 and T4.

In the **early stages of underactivity of the thyroid gland** it is often possible to get it to work normally again by taking **nutritional supplements** such as selenium, vitamin E, vitamin C, kelp and essential fatty acids. The thyroid gland has a high requirement for minerals, the most important ones being selenium, boron, iodine, zinc, magnesium, and manganese.

Selenium is vital for the conversion of T4 to the active T3 form and so will help those with thyroid resistance and excess weight due to underactivity of thyroid hormones.

If blood tests show that you are only in the very early stages of thyroid underactivity (hypothyroidism), these nutritional supplements may be enough to get the thyroid gland functioning normally again. This means you may be able to delay taking thyroid hormone tablets for some time. It is always best to be able to get your own glands functioning normally if possible, even if it is only for several years, rather than taking hormone tablets. You will need to be guided by your own doctor here, as in some people the failure of the thyroid gland is severe, in which case thyroid hormone is always needed along with nutritional medicine.

Give your cells the vital raw materials they need to manufacture hormones and enzymes and you should be able to restore normal cellular function.

In some people the thyroid gland becomes overactive and produces excessive amounts of thyroid hormone. This is called **hyperthyroidism** and may cause fatigue, anxiety, insomnia, tremor, muscle wasting and weakness, weight loss, palpitations, heart failure and other severe symptoms. The reason that the thyroid gland is pumping out excessive amounts of thyroid hormone in those with hyperthyroidism is because the gland is inflamed and irritated by something, such as a virus or abnormal antibodies. In this situation the immune system is overloaded and can be greatly helped with a liver-cleansing diet (see my *Liver-Cleansing Diet* book published in 1996). It is also vital to take anti-inflammatory supplements to calm down the hyped-up thyroid gland and I recommend anti-oxidants (vitamin E, C, selenium, magnesium and essential fatty acids). Those with an overactive thyroid gland must **not** take supplements containing iodine, such as kelp or seaweed. If the thyroid gland is very overactive drugs, such as neomercazole, will be required for a temporary period and during this time also use a liver-cleansing diet and the supplements to calm down the thyroid gland. You will need to see your doctor regularly.

In those troubled by thyroid cysts and lumps filled with mucous (multinodular goitre), the diet is very important and to shrink these cysts you will need to avoid mucous-forming foods such as dairy products, margarines, fatty meats and processed foods.

In patients with CFS it is important to check for an underactive thyroid gland. The thyroid gland is the body's throttle and regulates the speed of metabolism. It manufactures thyroxine known as T4 which is the storage form of thyroid hormone. The body has to convert this to the active form of thyroid hormone known as triidothyronine or T3. Most thyroid hormone medications are synthetic forms of T4, such as oroxine and only work effectively if your body can convert them into active T3. So it is important that your doctor measures both T4 and T3 levels. If this is not done, some people with underactive thyroid function will be missed. The mitochondria require T3 to burn oxygen and make the energy fuel called ATP for cells to function. With advancing years the body produces less T3 which may cause energy production in the mitochondria to become inadequate. By replacing both T4 and T3 in such cases, we can rejuvenate the mitochondria—our cellular furnaces—so that their production of ATP increases to normal levels. This restores our energy levels and slows down the ageing process.

If your thyroid gland is underactive (hypothyroidism) you will notice signs of a slowing down of metabolism. You will gain weight easily, be very tired, constipated and may feel excessively cold. Your skin will be dry and start to wrinkle and you hair will thin. Your cholesterol levels will start to go up because thyroid hormone plays a role in regulating fat metabolism. It is easy to attribute these symptoms to 'normal ageing', which is why it is so important to do tests for thyroid function.

TESTS FOR THYROID GLAND FUNCTION:

1. Blood level of T4.
2. Blood level of T3.
3. Blood level of thyroid stimulating hormone (TSH), which is made by the pituitary gland. If TSH is too high this means that the T4 and/or T3 levels are too low and that the pituitary gland is pumping out larger amounts of TSH to try to stimulate the thyroid gland into producing more T4.
4. Blood level of transthyretrin (prealbumin), which is a protein that transports thyroid hormone through the bloodstream. If this protein is too low it could mean that even if your thyroid gland is producing adequate thyroid hormone, it is not being taken to the cells.

Those with even a slight degree of thyroid underactivity usually feel a great boost to well-being after thyroid replacement therapy is begun. Usually synthetic T4 in the form of thyroxine is prescribed; however, it is wise to keep a check on T3 levels because if these do not come up to normal with thyroxine tablets, it is necessary to prescribe T3 hormone in the form of tertroxin tablets. In the USA a small number of doctors prescribe a desiccated thyroid product, which is animal based and was used before thyroxine and tertroxin became available. Desiccated thyroid products contain both T4 and T3, which some believe to be more natural than synthetic thyroid hormone. I have found that patients generally do very well on the synthetic forms of thyroid replacement and the dosage is easier to manipulate to fine-tune the blood levels of T4 and T3.

THE ADRENAL GLANDS

Another fascinating part of our glandular system is the set of two adrenal glands that sit like little 'hats' upon the top of each kidney. Their smallness belies their power, for these diminutive glands produce the potent hormones cortisone, dehydroepiandrosterone (DHEA for short!), and adrenalin. Indeed, the adrenal glands are programmed in tune with the body's circadian rhythm, so that they produce a surge of these energising hormones in the morning, to give us the stamina to face the challenges of the new day. Here comes a hint! If you do not feel well in the mornings and drag yourself out of bed, looking for coffee, sugar, cigarettes, and other stimulants, then your adrenal glands may be underactive. If they were working efficiently, their extra morning pulse of cortisone, DHEA and adrenalin would have you bouncing out of bed and raring to go. I have found that many people who suffer with chronic fatigue and/or morning depression have adrenal gland exhaustion. This is often the outcome of poor diet, heavy smoking, prolonged stress, chronic illness or recurrent viral infections. It is quite common in 'superwomen', who are high achievers or very caring, and yet never seem to get enough rest for themselves.

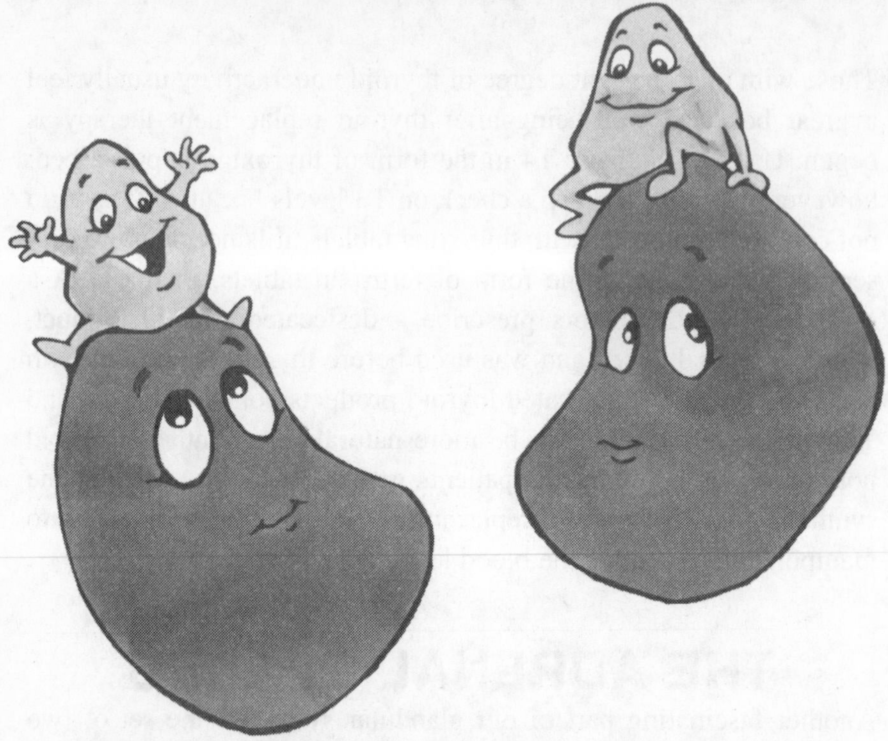

The adrenal glands sit like 'little hats' upon the top of each kidney—they produce energising hormones to give us the stamina to face the challenges of the new day.

If you have this adrenal burnout I suggest you rejuvenate your adrenal glands with our energy diet which is high in anti-oxidants and essential fatty acids. You will also need daily supplements of vitamin E, 1000 IU, vitamin C, 1000–2000 mg, vitamin B_5 (pantothenic acid), 200 mg, selenium, 200 mcg and magnesium chelates, 1000–2000 mg.

Essential fatty acids help the cortical cells of the adrenal gland which are found in its outer layer, called the adrenal cortex. Essential fatty acids can be found in evening primrose oil, flaxseed oil, oily fish, avocadoes and other seed oils. Sporty people and those who do aerobics will find their endurance and performance enhanced through boosting the adrenal glands. Many with morning depression will find that their moods improve after rejuvenating the adrenals with supplements.

Your adrenal glands can be checked with a blood test done both in the morning and in the late afternoon and this should reflect the normal boost in cortisone levels in the mornings. If the blood tests do not show this, you should find that the above supplements overcome this sluggish adrenal gland function.

Each adrenal gland consists of two parts. The centre of the gland makes the hormone called adrenalin, which enables the body's metabolism to speed up to cope with stressful situations. The outer layer of each adrenal gland is called the adrenal cortex and this makes several powerful hormones. These are:

1. Dehydroepiandrosterone (DHEA)

The adrenal cortex, if healthy, makes large amounts of DHEA, which promotes energy, sex drive and general well-being. Although DHEA levels normally decline with age, they reduce prematurely in many patients with chronic fatigue. These patients often respond dramatically to supplementation with DHEA.

2. Cortisol

This is also known as cortisone and is involved in the control of blood pressure and blood sugar levels, as well as immune function. If the adrenal cortisol production is insufficient the patient may feel very tired, suffer from excessive inflammation and allergies, low blood sugar levels, reduced immune function and very low blood pressure. They may feel extremely tired and depressed in the morning when the cortisol levels are too low.

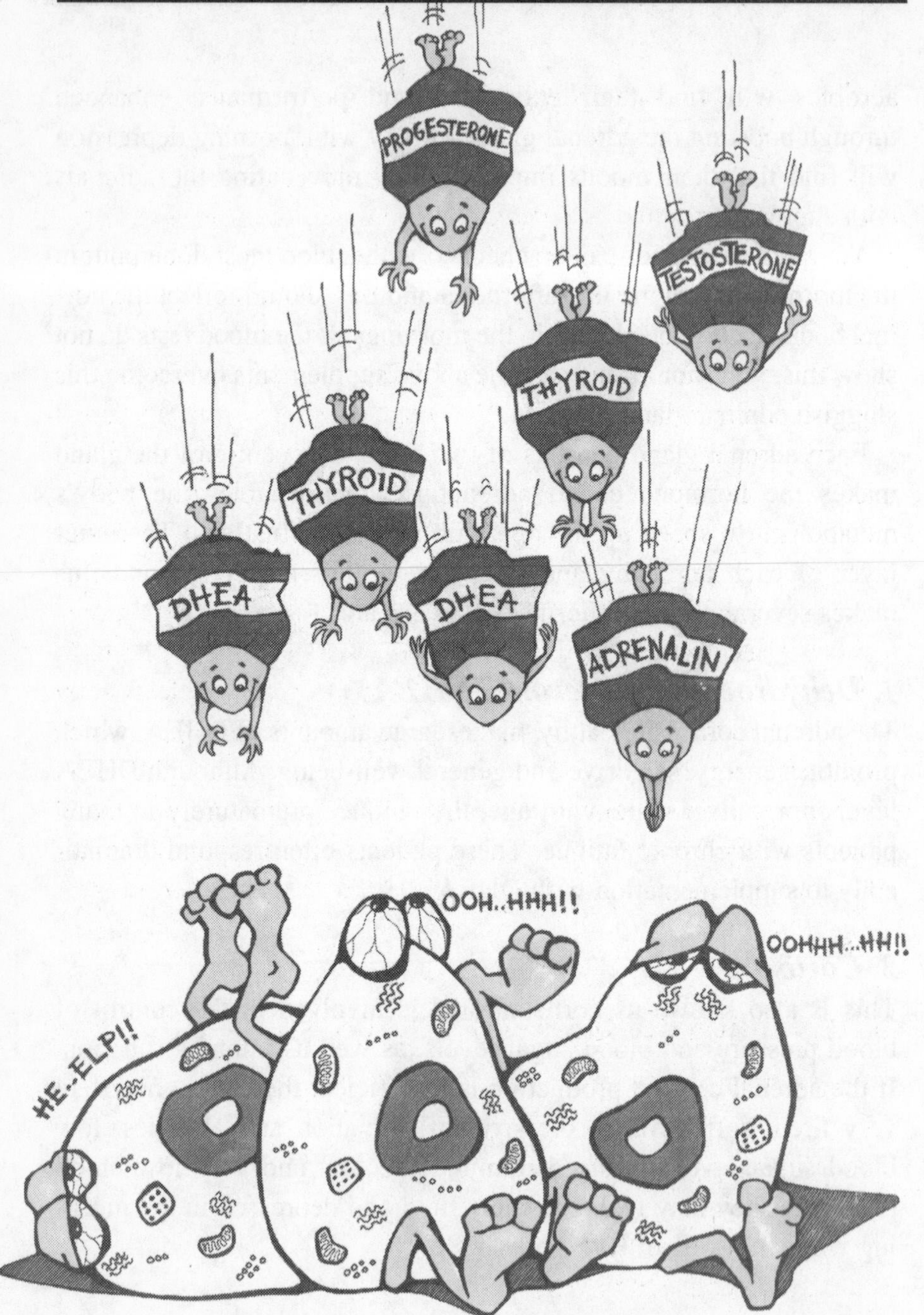

The superhormones rush to the rescue of ailing body cells.

3. Testosterone and Oestrogen

The adrenal cortex makes small amounts of these sex hormones which are also produced by the testicles and ovaries in larger amounts. During female menopause when the ovaries fail, the adrenal production of testosterone and oestrogen becomes much more important and takes over the role of the ovaries to a large degree. Thus, healthy adrenal glands are very important during the menopausal years and also during the years after menopause.

The technique of hormone replacement needs to be finely tuned during menopause, otherwise it may cause imbalances in the adrenal glands. For example, if excessive doses of potent oestrogen replacement is given, this may suppress the adrenal production of androgens, such as testosterone and DHEA. This can result in fatigue, depression and mood disorders. Every hormone that we give in hormone replacement therapy, be it oestrogen, testosterone, DHEA, progesterone, thyroid hormone etc., will cause a rebound effect upon our own glands. If excessive doses are used this will suppress our own glands too much, which will create new imbalances. This is why the technique of fine-tuning uses the smallest doses that are required of natural hormones in the correct combinations. It is like fine-tuning all the instruments in a symphony orchestra to create perfect harmony in the body.

Signs that your adrenal glands are underactive:

- Morning fatigue and depression
- General achiness
- Poor resistance to infections
- Inability to cope with stress
- Low blood pressure

- Low blood sugar levels
- Allergies
- Inflammatory problems
- Poor libido
- Dizziness

Modern medicine is realising that a person may feel unwell due to only mild to moderate deficiencies of hormones. In such cases blood tests may show hormone levels that are at the lower limits of the so-called 'normal range' of the general population. It is not necessarily in the patient's best interests to wait for a gland to fail almost completely, when its respective hormone level will fall below the bottom end of the normal scale. This may cause the patient to endure several years of poor health that could be avoided by rejuvenating the gland with nutritional supplements or, if this fails, by replacing the hormone to bring blood tests back into the middle levels of the normal range. Everyone is an individual and some people do not function well with hormone levels in the lower limits of the normal range. I have found that around 50 per cent of my patients with chronic fatigue have a slight but significant underactivity of their adrenal glands.

TESTS FOR ADRENAL GLAND FUNCTION

1. DHEA production

If DHEA levels are found to be low (less than 10 umol/l in males or less than 4 umol/l in females), this could indicate poor function of the adrenal cortex. A supplement of DHEA in a dose of 5–50 mg twice daily can be tried to bring blood DHEA levels into the middle of the normal scale for a person in their twenties. This will need to be fine-tuned regularly depending upon results of blood tests. We do not want to produce DHEA levels higher than 6 umol/l in a female or 13 umol/l in a male because side effects, such as acne or facial hair, may occur. Most patients feel well if their DHEA levels are not allowed to go below 4 umol/l.

2. Cortisol production

The most commonly performed test of adrenal gland function is the Synacthen Stimulation Test. This test checks the ability of the adrenal glands to pump out extra cortisol, when the glands are under stress. You can ask your doctor to do a Synacthen Stimulation Test if you suspect your adrenal glands are underactive. The test involves having an injection of another hormone called adrenocorticotrophic hormone (ACTH) and taking three separate blood samples to measure cortisol levels.

PATHWAYS OF HORMONE PRODUCTION

All steroid hormones (DHEA, cortisone, progesterone, oestrogen, testosterone, pregnenolone) are made in the body from the fat, cholesterol. Cholesterol is produced in the liver and is found in some foods, primarily dairy products and meat. Most people see cholesterol as a bad thing, associated with cardiovascular disease. It is true that excessively high levels of cholesterol are undesirable; however, very low levels of body cholesterol can also be unhealthy. This is because the body requires adequate cholesterol to produce steroid hormones, vitamin D and bile.

Cholesterol is also important for the function of the nervous system as it is used in the manufacture of myelin, which is the fatty layer

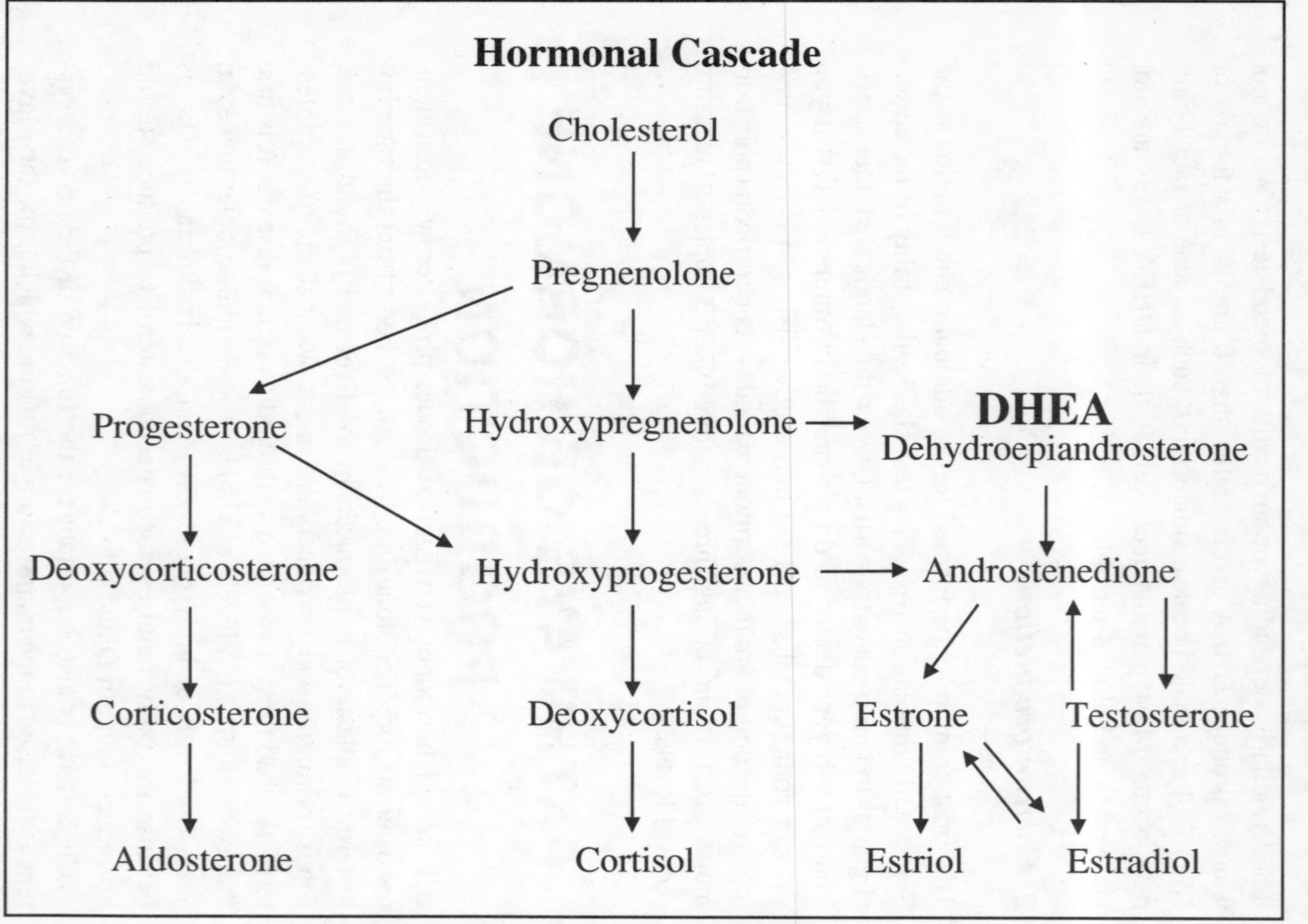

Biochemistry of the body's production of hormones.

surrounding the nerves. To produce steroid hormones cholesterol is first converted into a hormone called pregnenolone, which is then converted into other hormones in the steroid pathway (see diagram 34). Pregnenolone is like a reservoir or storage steroid hormone because it can be turned into progesterone or DHEA, depending upon the needs of the body.

Unfortunately, the ability of the body to convert cholesterol into pregnenolone declines with age, particularly around the time of menopause. Because pregnenolone is the source hormone for many other steroid hormones, the decline in its levels will result in a general decline in the levels of other hormones, such as DHEA, oestrogen, testosterone, progesterone and sometimes cortisone. Thankfully, replacement with pregnenolone is now available and this can help restore the overall balance of the body's steroid hormones, which is a very useful anti-ageing tool. This form of balancing must be prescribed by a medical doctor and regular follow-up is essential. This is because whenever any form of hormone replacement therapy is given it can produce hormonal or metabolic effects that vary from one individual to another and dosages must be carefully regulated.

DHEA

Your **DHEA** level is important because deficiency of this hormone has been implicated in chronic fatigue and premature ageing. DHEA (dehydroepiandrosterone) is made by the adrenal glands and is a 'mother' hormone or reservoir hormone, in that it is converted into other sex hormones, such as oestrogen and testosterone (see diagram page 34).

After the age of thirty, DHEA production progressively declines so that by the mid-seventies it's down to 20 per cent of its youthful peak. Also, during illness at any age, DHEA levels drop. I have found that the supplements recommended above for the adrenal glands can help DHEA production. For those with very low or non-detectable levels of DHEA, in association with severe fatigue, there may be a case for supplementing with the real DHEA hormone. This should be done by a medical doctor but, unfortunately, while DHEA is freely available in the USA, it is prohibited in Australia. Some studies have shown that DHEA can help with fatigue and premature ageing. (Reference 15).

Osteoporosis or age-related bone loss is another common problem likely to be helped by taking supplements of DHEA. We know that the sex steroids oestrogen and testosterone can reduce osteoporosis and, because DHEA is a source hormone for these other hormones (see diagram page 34), it should augment their bone-preserving effects. Giving DHEA to a group of post-menopausal women increased their levels of testosterone and oestrogens (Reference 16). DHEA has positive effects upon bone metabolism both directly and indirectly by increasing the levels of the hormones oestrogen and testosterone. During menopause, DHEA levels decline and this may be responsible for some menopausal symptoms, such as fatigue, depression and poor libido. A study found that average DHEA levels declined from 542 ng/100 ml in premenopausal women to 197 ng/100 ml in post-menopausal women. In women who had their ovaries surgically removed the average levels were only 126 ng/100 ml. Thus, supplementation with DHEA may be of benefit to women with very severe menopausal symptoms following the removal of their ovaries, who do not respond satisfactorily to oestrogen replacement alone. In a group of older women (55–85 years), it was found that those with lower levels of DHEA had lower bone density in their spines. This would predispose them to osteoporosis (Reference 17).

Dr William Regelson MD, from the Medical College of Virginia, believes that DHEA rejuvenates ageing immune systems by acting as a balancer for all adrenal hormones, including adrenal cortisone. This would make us more resilient to stress and increase endurance during times of mental and/or physical overload. Thus, it would be worthwhile for people with chronic fatigue syndrome, nervous overload and those who find that they no longer cope with stress as well as they did in their younger years. I must admit that I would feel more comfortable giving small amounts of DHEA to a patient with 'stress burnout' than I would giving sedative drugs. For people who find the years between fifty and one hundred fraught with stress and anxiety I believe that DHEA may in the near future provide a big improvement in the quality of their lives.

During the last several years an increasing number of American doctors have been giving DHEA to patients with chronic fatigue syndrome (CFS) whose blood levels of DHEA are below normal or in the low end of the normal range. Patients with CFS have often been ill for years and many never get well. In this context it is encouraging to see that some of these poor patients are finding an increase in energy levels and stamina after taking small to moderate doses of DHEA.

HOW MUCH DHEA DO YOU TAKE?

I think it is wise to have a blood test first to see what your level is. In Australia the normal adult ranges for DHEA are 2.2–9.1 umol/l in premenopausal women and 0.3–1.7 umol/l in post-menopausal women. American doctors who are expert in its use are recommending that patients should take the smallest amount needed to get their DHEA blood levels up into the middle to high levels of the normal young adult range.To achieve this they recommend between 50 to 200 mg daily in capsule form, or if you are using the lozenges (troches) the doses are much smaller, around 5 to 20 mg daily. This therapy is not cheap and is probably not for pensioners yet, at least not until it becomes an accepted medical treatment.

ARE THERE ANY RISKS TO DHEA?

DHEA is working wonders for millions of people, but it's early days yet. It is only over the last three years that people have been taking this hormone, so it is wise to be cautious and say that, honestly, we do not know at this time if taking the youth hormone DHEA for prolonged periods will have any, as yet unknown, side effects. However, it is a natural substance and provided people take the smallest necessary amount under medical supervision it should prove safe. Women with problems such as excessive body/facial hair, acne and balding due to excessive male hormones (androgens) will find that DHEA makes these problems worse. Overdosing on DHEA can increase your testosterone levels too much, causing facial hair and elevated cholesterol. So the technique of giving DHEA needs to be very finely tuned, using the smallest effective doses.

Men with andropause (male menopause) and/or chronic fatigue may benefit greatly from supplemental DHEA. However, men with prostate problems must be very cautious and only take DHEA after checking with their urologist. This is because any increase in testosterone is dangerous for men with prostate cancer or men who have high readings on prostate specific antigen (PSA) tests.

WHERE DO YOU GET DHEA?

Unfortunately, DHEA is not available in Australia because, quite surprisingly, it is considered an anabolic steroid by the authorities. If you go to America you will have no trouble finding it, as it is freely available on the shelves of health food stores. This is not good, as DHEA should only be prescribed by a medical doctor and dispensed by a compounding pharmacist, otherwise there is no quality control over what and how much people are taking

Many people will find it frustrating that DHEA is so hard to get in Australia and I can relate to that. It is frustrating! It should be available to those who really need it, provided it is controlled on a doctor's prescription. There are hundreds of drugs available in this country, including synthetic anabolic steroids, which are far more potent and potentially toxic than natural DHEA.

One of the reasons why DHEA is not easily available is that it is a natural hormone and, as such, it cannot be patented by drug companies for profit. This is also why drug companies do not fund huge clinical trials with DHEA and so ongoing research into its ability to retard ageing will continue relatively slowly. In fifteen to twenty years time the value of DHEA should be so obvious from the multitude of smaller independent researchers testing its effects, that worldwide medical authorities will be forced to accept it as a medical treatment of merit. However, twenty years will be too long for many older or sick people to wait.

In the meantime, you may want to find out about another natural adrenal hormone called pregnenolone, which has similar physiological effects to DHEA. For more information contact the Hormonal Advisory Service on (02) 4653 1445 or (02) 9387 8111.

PREGNENOLONE

Pregnenolone is a natural steroid hormone produced by the adrenal glands and, like all sex steroid hormones, it is made from cholesterol (see diagram 34).

Pregnenolone sits on top of the hormonal cascade and so, like DHEA, can be considered a mother hormone or reservoir for other sex steroid hormones. From DHEA and pregnenolone all the other steroid hormones are created, so we are talking about hormones that have very powerful balancing effects for those who need fine-tuning of the hormonal system.

Like DHEA, the levels of pregnenolone decrease with age from a peak around the mid-twenties down to the mid-seventies when levels become virtually non-detectable.

Pregnenolone was originally used as a treatment for inflammatory arthritis but when powerful synthetic steroidal anti-inflammatory drugs became available it was no longer used. A study published in the *Journal of the American Medical Association* way back in 1950, showed the beneficial effects of pregnenolone on rheumatoid arthritis without the side effects of synthetic steroids.

Recently, pregnenolone has been shown to be helpful for certain disorders of the central nervous system, such as memory loss, depression and fatigue. Pregnenolone can stimulate brain neuroreceptors by increasing glutamine uptake and can also calm the brain by activating GABA receptors. In this way pregnenolone regulates the emotional response and has a balancing effect upon the nervous system. People suffering from mood disorders and memory loss usually have low levels of pregnenolone in their cerebrospinal fluid (the fluid surrounding and bathing the brain). A study comparing healthy depression-free subjects with those who have chronic depression found that the depression-free individuals had double the level of pregnenolone (Reference 18). Studies have also found that as well as mood-enhancing properties, pregnenolone has the potential to improve memory. The US Air Force did studies on pregnenolone and found that it greatly reduced fatigue. It also found that after the pregnenolone was stopped, the reduction in fatigue lasted for about one month. Pregnenolone has been tested for many years as a treatment for arthritis and during this time has been found to be safe and free of side effects. It has been found to be helpful for mood disorders, memory loss and fatigue.

Theoretically, pregnenolone should also be helpful for many menopausal symptoms in men and women, such as loss of libido and fatigue and could be worth trying as a substitute for DHEA in these situations.

Pregnenolone is available only on prescription and is best taken in the form of hormonal troches (lozenges), which are placed between the gum and the cheek to slowly absorb into the bloodstream through the mucous lining of the cheek. These troches are best taken on an empty stomach in between meals. Dosage varies and a good starting dose is 50 mg daily for two months. If there is no improvement after this time, increase dosage to 100 mg daily for two months. Higher doses may be recommended by your doctor. If pregnenolone does not help you will need to consider other hormones, such as testosterone.

For more information contact the Hormonal Advisory Service in Sydney on (02) 46531445 or (02) 9387 8111 and speak to Beverley, Patricia or Jaqui and they can put you in touch with a compounding pharmacist.

THE SEX HORMONES

If you are a **premenopausal** woman you will probably notice that your energy levels fluctuate throughout the month and may be at their lowest during the week before menstrual bleeding. **Premenstrual fatigue** is aggravated by iron deficiency, unstable blood sugar levels and poor production from the ovary of the hormone progesterone. All of these things can be caused by poor diet and nutritional deficiencies.

I often call **progesterone** the **'happy hormone'** because it makes women feel relaxed and contented. Conversely, if the ovaries do not produce adequate amounts of progesterone you will be likely to feel tired, irritable, unmotivated and suffer with premenstrual syndrome (PMS). Lack of progesterone can also cause heavy painful menstrual bleeding and infertility. To help your ovaries produce more of this wonderful fertility hormone you need to ensure that you get plenty of vitamin E and essential fatty acids. Also, change your diet to increase phytoestrogens (plant hormones), which come from plants (vegetables and fruit), legumes (beans, peas, lentils, sprouts), seeds, berries and raw nuts. If your menstruation is heavy you may

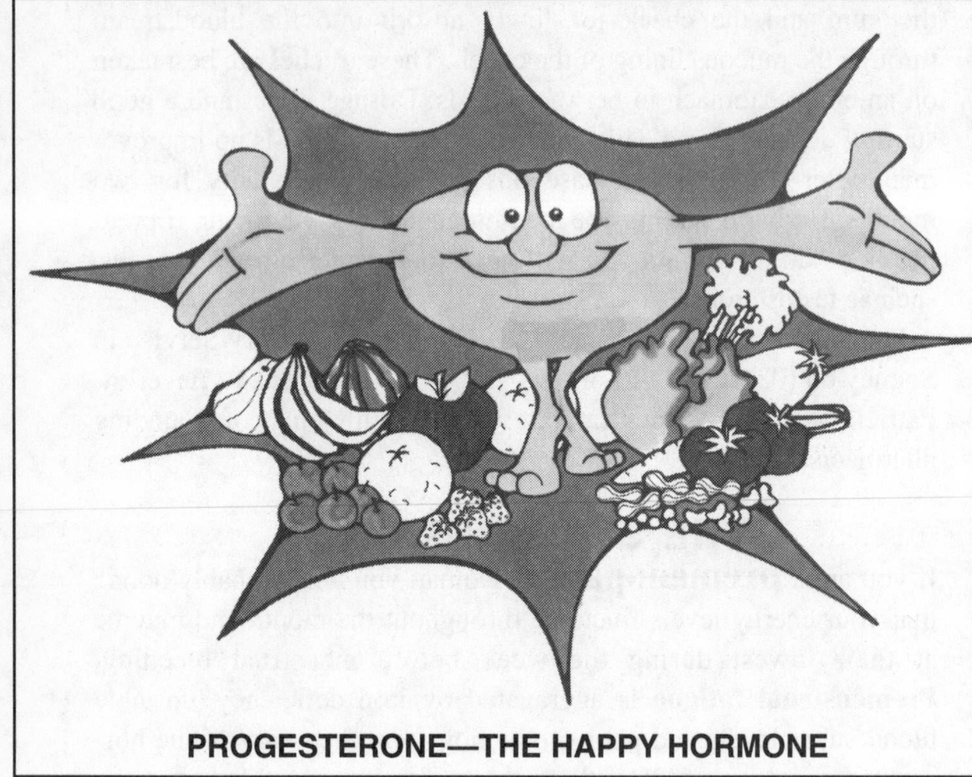

PROGESTERONE—THE HAPPY HORMONE

be iron deficient, which is easy to check with a blood test. Iron deficiency is one of the most common causes of chronic fatigue and can be helped with supplements of organic iron and spirulina.

Vitamin K (found in oily fish and dark green leafy vegetables) will often reduce heavy menstrual bleeding. A good way to boost your vitamin K and chlorophyll levels is with a raw fresh juice of spinach, beetroot greens and beetroots. This will give you a real energy boost and reduce heavy bleeding, especially if you stir in some spirulina powder. You may add apples to this juice to sweeten it if desired. To boost production of progesterone you will also need to increase your intake of essential fatty acids from evening primrose oil, flaxseed oil, fish oil and other cold-pressed seed oils. Most women will find that the above strategies overcome **premenstrual fatigue.** If, after three

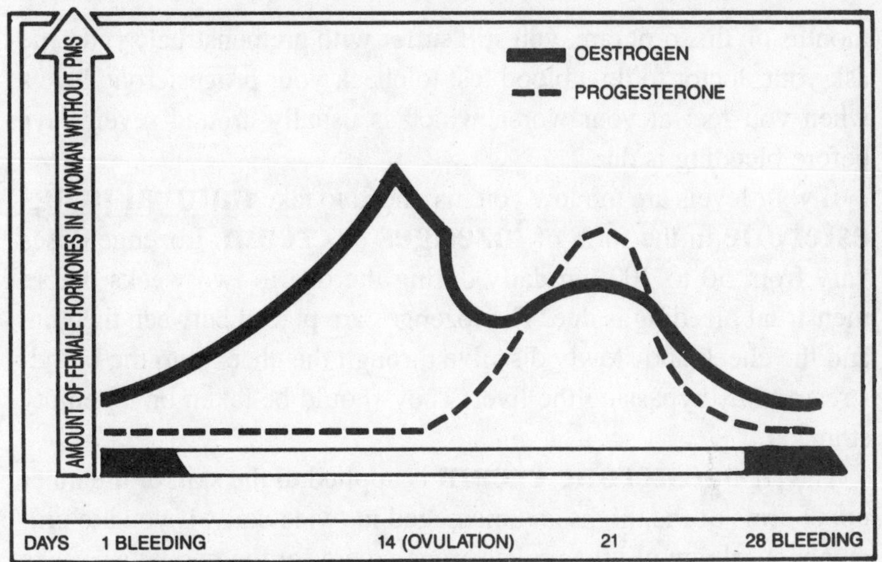

NORMAL MENSTRUAL CYCLE — WITHOUT PMS

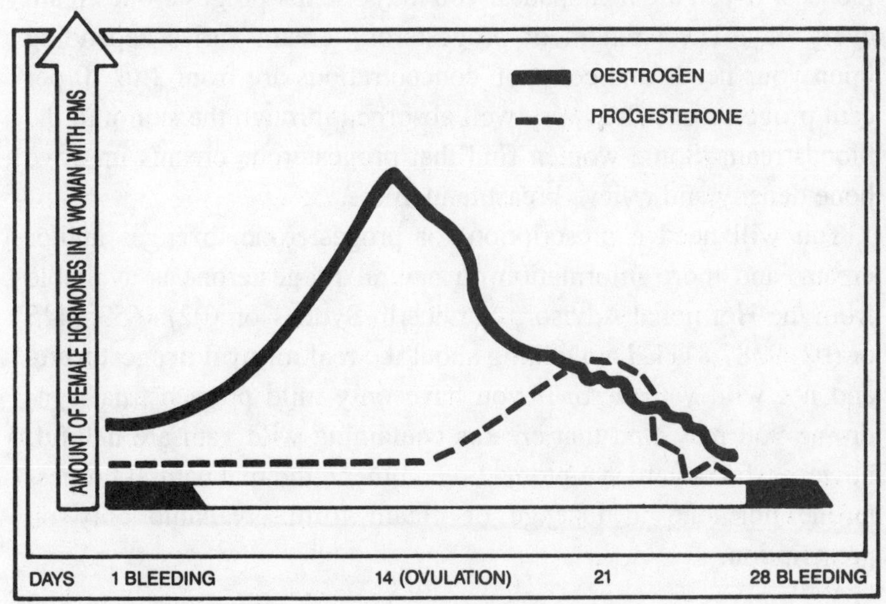

PMS=Premenstrual Syndrome

MENSTRUAL CYCLE — WITH PMS

months on this program, you still suffer with premenstrual syndrome ask your doctor to do a blood test to check your progesterone levels when you feel at your worst, which is usually around seven days before bleeding is due.

If your levels are too low you may need to take **natural progesterone** in the form of **lozenges** or **cream.** Lozenge doses vary from 50 to 200 mg daily during the one to two weeks before menstrual bleeding is due. The lozenges are placed between the gum and the cheek and slowly dissolve through the cheek into the bloodstream, thus bypassing the liver. They should be taken on an empty stomach.

The **progesterone cream** is applied to the skin of the inner upper arms or the thighs and massaged in twice daily. If you are premenopausal you use the progesterone cream for the two latter weeks of the menstrual cycle and stop when menstrual bleeding commences. If you are menopausal you may use the progesterone cream every day. The strength of progesterone cream varies depending upon your needs and common concentrations are from 2 to 10 per cent progesterone. It is very well absorbed through the skin into the bloodstream. Some women find that progesterone creams improve bone density and relieve breast tenderness.

You will need a prescription for progesterone lozenges and/or cream, and more information on natural progesterone is available from the Hormonal Advisory Service in Sydney on (02) 4653 1445 or (02) 9387 8111. I am talking about the real **natural progesterone** and not wild yam herb. If you have only mild premenstrual syndrome you may find that creams containing wild yam are helpful; however, for severe symptoms I recommend the real natural progesterone hormone in lozenge or cream form, available only on prescription.

PERIMENOPAUSE

If you are in the **perimenopausal age group** (40–60) and finding that you are excessively tired, I suggest you ask your doctor to do a blood test to check your levels of the sex hormones oestrogen, testosterone and progesterone. When checking the **male hormones** (androgens) it is important to check the level of the **free androgens,** for these are the active hormones that will determine how you feel. The best test for the free male hormones is the free androgen index (FAI). If the FAI is very low you may suffer with chronic fatigue, low libido, panic attacks, muscle weakness and wasting, bone loss and depression.

Thankfully we now have the **hormone troches (lozenges)** that can be **tailor-made** to contain just about any combination of sex hormones for your hormone replacement therapy. The other wonderful thing about these new hormone troches is that they can provide you with a much smaller dose of testosterone (male hormone) than was ever possible before. Using these small doses every day we can fine-tune the body and restore physiological amounts of sex hormones so that overdosage does not occur. In this way you can feel a tremendous improvement to your well-being without the side effects.

Many menopausal women with chronic fatigue and low sex drive have found that daily doses of testosterone, as small as 0.5–3 mg, are sufficient to make them feel energised and sexual again. For me, as a doctor trying to help menopausal women, this is such a relief, because as recently as twelve months ago the only form of testosterone available was in the form of injections or implants or synthetic tablets. These forms of testosterone were too potent for some women causing side effects such as weight gain, body and facial hair, deepening of the voice, greasy skin and hair and acne. They often produced an on/off effect, where you would feel like a superwoman for several weeks or months, only to be let down with a big bang once the hormones were used up by your body. Thus, the possibility of fine-tuning the hormones was very difficult—more like 'a bull in a china shop' approach. With the troches or lozenges small doses are provided to the body every day so that constant levels are maintained without over or under dosage occurring.

In women who have had a **premature menopause** (before the age of forty), or had their ovaries removed, implants of oestrogen and testosterone may be of great value, as these women may need higher doses than those which can be provided by the troches. Once again, every woman is an individual and some trial and error may be required.

Troches containing natural testosterone can also be used to treat men with symptoms of **male menopause**. This is called **'andropause'.** Men with this problem have abnormally low levels of androgenic hormones such as testosterone and DHEA in their bodies. This can produce symptoms, such as depression, fatigue, loss of muscle mass, loss of drive, loss of confidence and poor libido. In other words the warrior man turns into a mouse. Not good for the ego or self-esteem, not to mention the love life.

In the past, male menopause has been treated with hormone injections, implants or synthetic tablets which are relatively potent and tend to have an on/off effect. In other words they give a big burst of energy but they wear off with a bang and you are back to square one. With the troches a man can take small to moderate doses of natural testosterone every day, thus maintaining constant blood levels of testosterone giving a more balanced effect.

Even if a man decides to try the troches, it is still necessary to have a check up of the prostate gland from a urologist first to exclude prostate disease. Do not neglect this because prostate cancer is very common. Prostate cancer is much less common in men who have a diet high in anti-oxidants and phytoestrogenic foods (see page 64).

OESTROGEN

Troches can also be tailor-made to contain varying amounts of the **three natural oestrogens** (oestradiol, oestrone and oestriol) produced by the body. The proportions of each type of oestrogen required is determined by the patient's symptoms and age. Women with severe symptoms of oestrogen deficiency such as vaginal dryness, loss of libido, hot flushes and wrinkling will usually require the more potent oestrogen called oestradiol. Those with mild symptoms will find that the weaker forms of natural oestrogen, called oestrone and/or oestriol, are usually sufficient. Once again, very small doses may be used for those women who tend to get side effects from oestrogen replacement.

Long-term oestrogen replacement (for more than five years) may increase the risk of breast cancer and some women may not want to accept this risk. Some menopausal women stay on high doses of oestrogen replacement for too long, which may increase the risk of breast and uterine cancer. I do not personally prescribe potent oestrogens for older women (over fifty-five) in whom I encourage the use of only small doses of the weaker oestrogens, oestrone and oestriol. Older women, particularly those over sixty, often find the weaker forms of oestrogen much more suitable and also safer. As women get older the risk of breast cancer continues to climb, whether they take hormone replacement therapy or not. However, you do not want to be taking anything that could further increase your risk of breast cancer and this is one good reason to use smaller doses of weaker oestrogens as you get older, to relieve your menopausal symptoms.

Regular or average starting doses of oestradiol are from 1 to 2 mg daily. Some women feel better if they take all three oestrogens combined in one troche and a typical prescription for starting would be oestradiol 1 mg, oestrone 1 mg and oestriol 1 mg. If it is desired to use only a very small amount of oestrogen, a troche could be made up consisting of only oestrone 0.5 mg and oestriol 0.5 mg. Any

The symptoms that are characteristic of oestrogen deficiency may be grouped together in a chart and scored according to the following scale:

Absent = 0 Mild = 1 Moderate = 2 Severe = 3

TABLE 5: OESTROGEN LEVEL SCORE CHART

OESTROGEN DEFICIENCY SYMPTOM	SCORE (0-3)
Depression and mood changes	
Anxiety and/or irritability	
Unloved or unwanted feelings	
Poor memory and concentration	
Poor sleeping patterns (insomnia)	
Fatigue	
Backache	
Joint pains, increase in arthritis	
Muscle pains	
New facial hair	
Dry skin and/or sudden wrinkling	
Crawling, itching, burning sensations in the skin	
Reduced sexual desire	
Frequency or burning of urination	
Discomfort during sexual intercourse	
Vaginal dryness	
Hot flushes and/or excessive sweating	
Light-headedness or dizziness	
Headaches	
YOUR TOTAL SCORE:	

This chart is derived from Professor Nordin's Menopause Questionnaire, Institute of Medical & Veterinary Science, Adelaide, South Australia.

If your total score for all of these symptoms is 15 or more, then it is likely that you are suffering with a deficiency of oestrogen. If your score is around 30, your body is crying out for oestrogen. This can be confirmed or refuted with a simple blood test to check your level of oestrogen and Follicle Stimulating Hormone.

It is an interesting exercise to score your symptoms of oestrogen deficiency before and after commencing Hormone Replacement Therapy.

combination is possible and it may take some trial and error using different combinations in different amounts over several months before the ideal combination is found. The body produces the three natural oestrogens in the following proportions—oestriol 80 per cent, oestradiol 10 per cent, oestrone 10 per cent and this is available as a hormone product called Triest that may be put into a troche. Some women like to use the combination of oestrogens found in Triest because it is closest to their own body's natural production of oestrogen. However, this is not essential as other women may want to use more or less of the stronger oestrogen, oestradiol.

The beauty of the troches is their flexibility and if your troche is too strong you can simply cut it in half or quarters to save money and avoid side effects. Of course, you will need to do this under your own doctor's supervision.

Your own doctor should be able to advise you on the safety of oestrogen in your particular case. I would advise you to avoid oestrogen replacement completely or only use very small doses of the weaker oestrogens if you have tender lumpy breasts or a strong family history of breast cancer. Very small daily doses of the weaker oestrogens would be oestrone 0.2 to 0.5 mg or oestriol 0.2 to 0.5 mg in troche form. These weaker oestrogens can also be put into a cream, either by themselves or combined with natural progesterone and/or testosterone. These creams can be rubbed into the skin of the vulva, vagina or buttocks and inner thighs once or twice daily.

The **oestrogen patches** are also very useful because they bypass the liver and provide a relatively low dose of oestrogen. They are much safer in women with medical problems, such as heart disease, high blood pressure, varicose veins, fluid retention, liver and gall bladder problems, migraine headaches and obesity. The patches are also very flexible because they come in many different doses which enables you and your doctor to mix and match until you find the right dose for you.

Estraderm patches are available in 3 sizes.

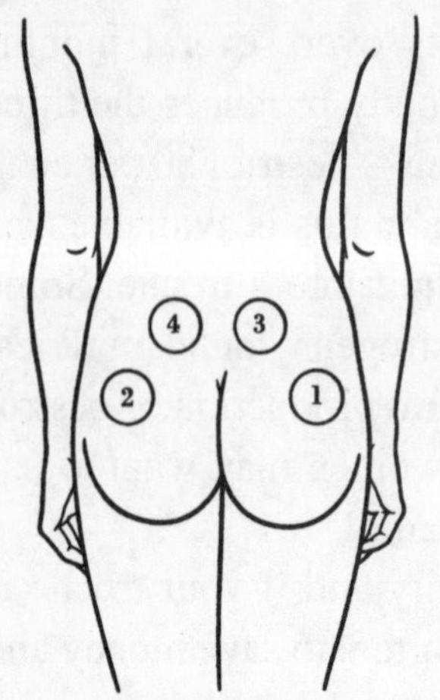

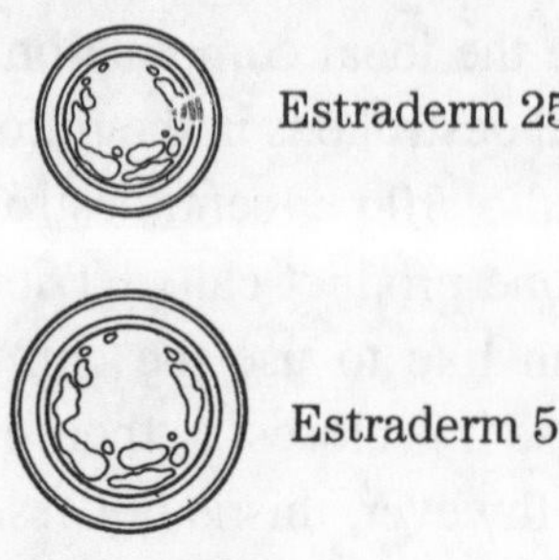

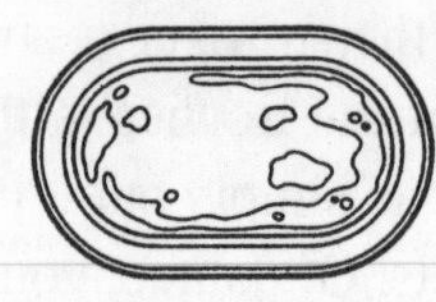

Suggested application sites of Estraderm patches:

1 & 2 first week
3 & 4 second week
1 & 2 third week etc

Women who are worried about **breast cancer** can use lozenges or creams containing **only** progesterone and perhaps a small amount of testosterone, along with phytoestrogens (see page 64) as their hormone replacement therapy.

Women who are carrying **excessive weight** may have sufficient oestrogen and testosterone levels even after menopause, as these hormones are produced by the fat cells. However, they may have a deficiency of progesterone which is causing fatigue and menstrual disturbances. In such women only natural progesterone is required in the form of troches or creams along with phytoestrogens (see page 64).

I have found that women of the 'android body type' (see page 51) often put on weight in the upper part of the body around the chest and abdomen, when they get into the perimenopausal years.

Android women (and men), put on weight very easily around the midriff in middle age because they tend to have a dysfunctional liver. I have noticed that the condition of 'fatty liver' is more common in android body types and may be associated with excess weight gain, high cholesterol, high blood pressure and non-insulin dependent diabetes. In such cases, we do not want to give high

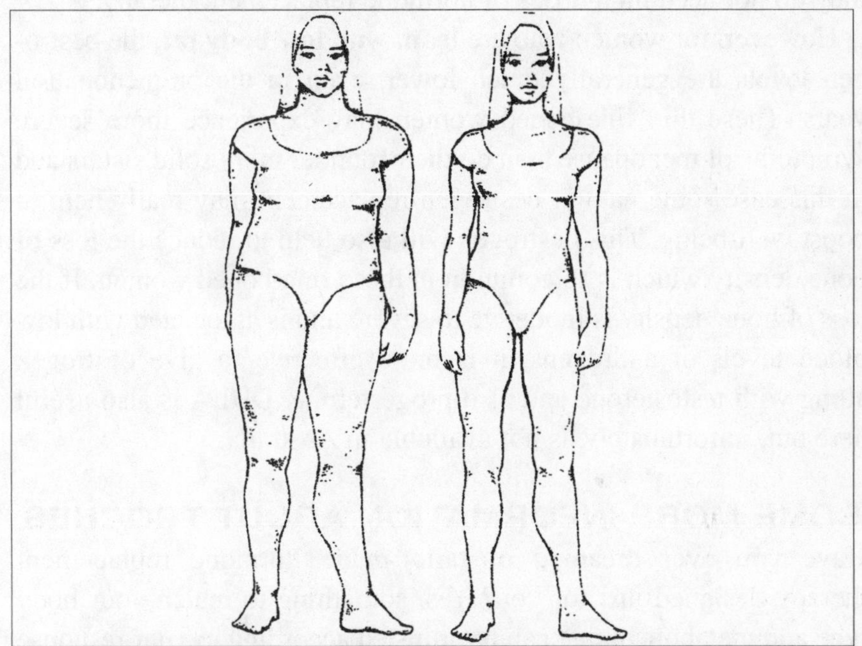

Android body shape (left) overweight, (right) ideal weight.

doses of any hormones, particularly oestrogen and/or testosterone, as this will only overload the liver further and lead to more weight gain and fatigue. It may also elevate the blood pressure and increase cardiovascular problems. Indeed, overweight android women generally do much better with only phytoestrogens. If hormone replacement therapy is used the best choices are patches or very low dose troches.

If hormone replacement therapy is given inappropriately it will not reduce cardiovascular disease.

Android women often have good levels of natural testosterone production and sometimes their natural oestrogen levels are also quite good, even after menopause. They also tend to have big bones, with a high bone density, so their risk of osteoporosis is not high. Thus, they do not need high doses of hormone replacement therapy.

However, for women who are **lean,** with **low body fat,** the oestrogen levels are generally much lower, even in the premenopausal years. These thin fine-boned women may experience more severe symptoms of menopause than do their rounder more solid sisters and in this case some natural oestrogen replacement may really help to boost well-being. This oestrogen will also help to reduce the loss of bone density which is so common in these fine-boned women. If the loss of bone density is moderate to severe and is associated with low blood levels of androgens, it is more effective to give oestrogen along with testosterone and also progesterone. DHEA is also useful here but, unfortunately, is not available in Australia.

SOME MORE INFORMATION ABOUT TROCHES

Have you ever dreamed of tailor-made hormone replacement therapy designed just for you? Yes, something to match your body type and metabolism that can be adjusted according to your response over time so that side effects and efficacy can be controlled easily. This is the concept of fine-tuning and it is now possible because of troches. Troches are small square lozenges that are placed between the gum and the cheek. They slowly dissolve through the mucous lining of the cheek into the bloodstream, largely bypassing the liver. They have been available in Australia for one year, from a compounding chemist in Sydney. Prior to this they were only available from America at considerable expense. This is a breakthrough for the thousands of women who find that prescriptions for commercially packaged hormone replacement therapy are too strong or produce too many side effects.

Troches can be mixed so that each individual troche contains a combination of various natural hormones in small doses. For example, a troche can be made containing a mixture of any of the hormones oestrogen, progesterone, pregnenolone and/or testosterone in any possible doses according to your symptoms and the results of your blood tests. Small doses of testosterone can be used, such as 1–2 mg per troche, so that masculinising side effects, such as facial hair, acne, weight gain and voice deepening, are avoided. This provides a much more gentle approach than injections or implants of testosterone or indeed the synthetic testosterone tablets that have been used in the past. Small doses of testosterone and/or pregnenolone are useful to enhance energy levels, mood and libido, without causing side effects.

Troches containing pure natural progesterone are helpful for premenstrual syndrome, premenstrual tension, pelvic congestion or postnatal depression. For emotional problems caused by hormonal imbalance they are far superior to tablets containing synthetic progesterones which are known as progestagens.

Menopausal women who have had a hysterectomy can benefit from troches containing natural oestrogens, progesterone and, if needed, testosterone. Your requirements should be determined with a blood test to measure your sex hormones. I recommend tests for blood oestrogen, progesterone and testosterone (free androgen index or FAI).

Compounding pharmacist, Richard Stenlake tells us that pharmacy is going 'back to the future'. We are now using century-old techniques to create custom-tailored medicines for a growing percentage of doctors and their patients. We are creating medications from scratch or altering existing medications to meet specific patient needs. This technique goes back to the original apothecaries of the 1800s who made every prescription by hand. This practice gradually faded from use as pharmaceutical companies began mass producing drugs in set doses and patients had to contend with whatever dose was closest to what they needed.

Back in the 1800s, medical lozenges were used extensively to treat mouth and throat infections. These were small mildly medicated solid masses intended to dissolve in the mouth. In England they were called a lozenge, in the USA, a troche, in France, a tab lette and, in Germany, a pastillen. Troches first appeared in the *Edinburgh Pharmacopoeia* in 1841 and in the *British Pharmacopoeia* in 1864—the same book is the gold standard of today's pharmacists.

Troche making was an art way back then and required a lot of practical experience. The apparatus required to make troches was a smooth marble slab to mix them, a rolling pin, troche cutters, a palette knife, a brush with long soft hairs, linen cloth and troche trays. Yes, the apothecary of the early nineteenth century required great skill to make this form of medication. This art was still taught at universities until the late 1960s when the twentieth century really took over. The theory of troche and pill making was still taught but, sadly, practical knowledge was left to a bygone age. One could compare the mass-produced drugs of today with fast convenience foods and the troches to carefully prepared home-cooked meals!

The troches provide a means to deliver custom-made medication in small doses directly into the bloodstream. Today, many drugs, both natural and synthetic, can be used in troche form to gain rapid onset of action and bypass the usual absorption through the small intestines. This reduces the load upon the liver and is especially good for liver-toxic drugs.

Through technology from the Professional Compounding Centres of America (PCCA), troches are now a modern-day dosage form, available in a variety of bases and flavours that the apothecary of old could not even imagine. There is still an art in compounding them but the equipment required has greatly diminished.

Today, the computer has replaced the marble slabs, the wooden trays and brushes. There are complex electronic mixers, mint-flavoured bases, accruable electronic scales (capable of measuring much less than milligram doses) and miniature electric hot plates that make the finished troches an accurate precise dosage form. The finished troches are dispensed in plastic calibrated moulds that fit easily into your handbag. The flavours available from the PCCA now cover over three pages and can satisfy even the most finicky patient. How would you like peanut butter, creme de menthe, toffee, kahlua?—to name a few of the more exotic. You can try a different flavour every month to prevent hormonal boredom!

Troches are very well suited to hormone replacement therapy for both men and women, mainly because of the ease in which ingredients in each prescription can be altered. As troches are made up in trays of only twenty-four, you will know after one or two courses if the prescription is correct for you, or is a little off the mark. By this we mean that there could be a little too much/too little progesterone or too much/too little oestrogen. After a quick consultation with your doctor, the formula can be altered and your medication tailor-made to your exact requirement. Compare this to mass-produced drugs where individual titration of doses is far more limited.

Compounding a medication imparts to the pharmacist a greater stake in the patient's outcome. The pharmacist keeps in close contact with the patient, enabling early identification of the patient's needs and any side effects. This allows the pharmacist to use his/her skills to overcome problems through consultation with both patient and doctor to produce the correct dosage form that will result in long-term success.

HORMONAL TRUTH

For well over twenty years I have been researching the area of hormonal medicine, the specialty of which is called endocrinology. Through my own medical practice and health seminars, which I have conducted all over the world, I have seen many thousands of women who suffer from hormonal problems. Sometimes I laugh when people ask me if I have been through menopause and I often reply, 'Yes I have, not just once, but thousands of times along with my patients!'

As you can imagine, when I first began trying to help women with hormonal problems such as premenstrual syndrome, postnatal depression and menopause, the treatments available were very limited. There was virtually no information available to women with these problems and women generally suffered in silence. I studied and read medical journals profusely and yet the material I found was usually too esoteric and academic and not of much practical help to women out there in the suburbs who were pulling their hair out. Most of the research was being done by men who lived in academic ivory towers and had never lived with the mighty force of a hormonal depression.

Over the last twenty years this has all changed and there is now a plethora of books available on hormonal problems, some of them with sensational titles that read like a 'days of our lives' novel. Some are written by non-medical persons who have never had the experience of trying to help women with hormonal problems. These people write vicariously having had no hands-on experience to prove their theories. Some of these books describe one single hormone or herb as the panacea to good health for all hormonal women and intimate that what regular doctors are doing is dangerous. They paint a simplistic picture and usually put all women into the same category, saying that they are all being poisoned and should all change to product X. You may find that these books are a vehicle for promoting product X. Yes, sensationalism does sell but, unfortunately, it also confuses those with poor health and hormonal imbalance who are looking for a solution.

In all sincerity I wish that it was that simple and by taking product X we could all achieve hormonal equanimity. During my long career in helping women with hormonal upheaval I have found that it is not that black and white. Indeed, many things in medicine are not black and white. This is because patients are all individuals with unique hormonal and metabolic characteristics. What suits one patient will not always be correct for another and herein lies the challenge of good medicine and fine-tuning every individual. It is easy to give every hormonally imbalanced woman the same prescription for product X, while it is much harder to spend the time doing blood tests, bone-density tests, thorough physical examinations and taking a good history to determine what the individual requires for hormonal balancing.

There are many pressures on women today that come from society and the media in all its forms. Remember that the media like to tell sensational stories and don't always give you a balanced view of new health information. Some women are made to feel that menopause is a disease and that they must take hormones to keep them young and ward off Alzheimer's disease. The menopause is a multi-million dollar industry and there is a lot of money to be made pushing all types of hormones—both synthetic and natural. In this hormonal storm, do not get frightened but work with your own doctor to determine if you really need to take hormone therapy and make sure that you get the best type for your individual requirements and not just what is in vogue at the time.

There is a particular theory around at the moment called 'oestrogen dominance' which is used to describe the sea of synthetic oestrogens that women are currently drowning in. This theory goes on to say that the great majority of hormonally imbalanced women need progesterone and not oestrogen. This theory is far too simplistic and confuses women. The truth is, that most of the oestrogens used for menopause are natural and can be given in many forms to bypass the liver if required. Furthermore, very small physiological doses of oestrogen can be used. Remember, it is oestrogen that makes you a woman and gives you a female figure, vaginal lubrication, nice skin and a feminine appearance. Progesterone on the other hand is mainly required for fertility and to balance the effect of oestrogen upon the uterus. Progesterone may have other benefits, such as a calming effect, a bone-building effect and the reduction of breast and uterine cancer. Yes, these are important effects but not enough to negate the benefit of oestrogen replacement for many menopausal women, especially those with severe symptoms, osteoporosis, rapid ageing and sexual problems. Amid all the confusion remember that oestrogen is the primary female hormone that gives you your female characteristics and makes you look and feel like a woman. If given correctly, oestrogen can also reduce the risk of cardiovascular disease. For those women who go through a premature menopause and those fine-boned women with osteoporosis, progesterone alone may not be enough. In this situation best results are often achieved by a mixture of hormones, as determined by blood tests, with oestrogen and testosterone being beneficial.

I am also asked a lot of questions about creams made from the herb wild yam and many women ask me if this cream is enough to treat their menopause. These women have often been frightened off taking any form of hormone replacement therapy for fear of increasing their risk of cancer. My response is that, once again, every woman is an individual. For menopausal women with mild symptoms and good bone density, wild yam cream may be all that you need. I personally prefer to use wild yam with other phytoestrogenic herbs, such as black cohosh, dong quai and liquorice (see page 61), as then you are getting the full spectrum of herbal oestrogens. Wild yam contains the plant hormone diosgenin, which can be converted into progesterone in the laboratory. Just how efficiently the body turns the diosgenin in wild yam into progesterone is not known.

Learn to listen to your own body, it will tell you if something is working or not. Generally, hormonal treatments take four to eight weeks to fully exert their effects, so if you are not feeling any better after this time you are on the wrong track.

I think that today many women trying to ease their hormonal imbalances suffer with information overload and are uncertain what is the best path to follow. Remember that menopause is not a disease and relax, as there is no urgency. In this book I have tried to give you the true facts about all your hormonal options without any sensationalism or predjudice. I am not pushing any particular treatment as there are different courses for different horses.

I am not trying to be politically correct to fit in with the established thoughts, practises and philosophies of the day because many of these viewpoints are coloured by large amounts of funding, drug companies, bureaucracies and individuals in high places who wield enormous power over the collective thought processes. What I have presented you with is my perspective, based upon years of treating many difficult cases and corresponding with medical researchers at the cutting edge of independent research.

If some do not agree with me, this is good because new ideas that provoke lateral thought and challenge old limitations will get people talking and asking questions. We should always be trying to learn more and be willing to listen to our patients because they will teach us just as much as the text books and universities.

CHAPTER FOUR

PHYTOESTROGENS

The word **'phytoestrogens'** means **plant hormones.** Many foods, plants and some herbs contain plant hormones which can be used by humans to enhance health and regulate hormones. Phytoestrogens are able to mimic the effects of human oestrogens because their chemical structure is very close to that of human oestrogen. The better known phytoestrogen compounds are isoflavones, flavones and lignans. As women age and their natural production of oestrogen diminishes, phytoestrogens become more important and to some degree take over the role of ovarian oestrogens. Thus, phytoestrogens can have an anti-ageing effect.

There is a large amount of research going on all over the world into the effects of phytoestrogens upon the symptoms of menopause. It is fascinating that orthodox medicine is finally starting to scrutinise and accept the ancient teachings of European naturopaths and Chinese herbalists. It really shows us the circle of life, with modern-day thinking returning to the beginning of ancient teachings.

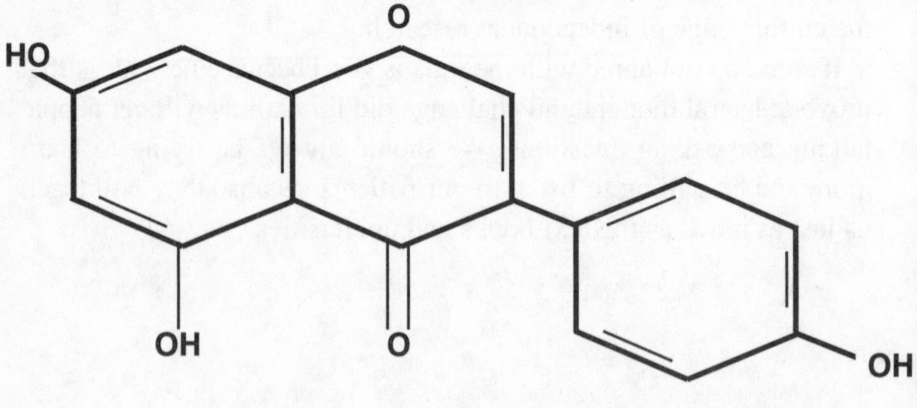

Structure of phytoestrogen.

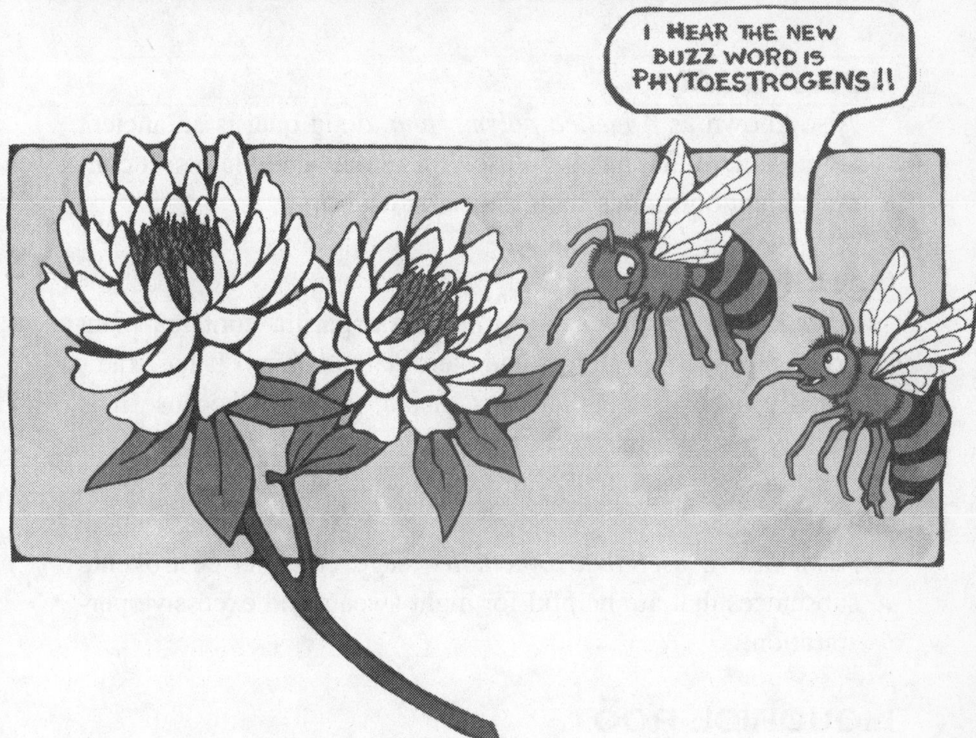

So the **buzz word** is PHYTOESTROGENS and people are starting to spread the word; however, women are confused because they don't know where to find these beneficial hormones.

PHYTOESTROGENS ARE FOUND IN THE FOLLOWING HERBS:

BLACK COHOSH

Also known as *Cimicifuga racemosa,* black cohosh is a native plant of North America and was used by the American Indians to treat fatigue and female disorders.

DONG QUAI

Also known as *Angelica polymorpha,* dong quai is an ancient Chinese herb that has been used for female complaints. It contains plant hormones such as beta-sitosterol.

SARSPARILLA ROOT

Also known as *Smilax officinalis,* sarsparilla contains plant hormones such as sterols and steroidal saponins. It has traditionally been used as an aphrodisiac, probably because it is slightly testosteronal.

SAGE

Also known as *Salvia officinalis,* sage contains oestrogenic substances that are helpful for night sweats and excessive perspiration.

LIQUORICE ROOT

Also known as *Glycyrrhiza glabra,* liquorice contains phytoestrogens that exert a balancing effect upon oestrogenic activity. It can also act as a tonic for those with morning fatigue due to adrenal gland exhaustion.

WILD YAM

Also known as *Dioscorea,* wild yam has been popularised by the many brands of wild yam creams used to treat premenstrual syndrome. Wild yam contains the hormone diosgenin which is similar in structure to the adrenal hormone DHEA. Diosgenin may have a balancing effect upon the body's hormones similar to the effect of DHEA and progesterone, although much weaker. Wild yam can help to overcome the negative effects of declining levels of DHEA and progesterone that occur with ageing. Wild yam can help those with fatigue, depression and loss of sex drive. I find it is more effective if taken orally and combined with other phytoestrogen herbs.

Other useful herbs for **perimenopausal** women are **kelp** and **horsetail** as their high mineral content is good for the bones, hair and thyroid gland.

PHYTOESTROGEN MIXTURES

All these herbs can be taken individually but it is much more effective and economical to take them all combined together (with vitamins, minerals, soy protein, linseed and alfalfa) in powder or capsule form. The dosage is one teaspoon of powder stirred into fruit juice, twice daily or two capsules twice daily just **before** food. In this form you are providing your body with a total hormonal and nutritive food, a type of 'superfood' for menopause, that can help all the menopausal symptoms. By combining all these things, you are supplying your bones, hair, skin and immune system with strengthening nutrients as well as phytoestrogens. I have found that powders containing a mixture of phytoestrogen herbs, foods and minerals are a good source of trace elements for the bones. If you rely on using only one herbal or food source of phytoestrogens, you will be missing out on the full spectrum of benefits obtainable from using a combination of the herbs I have discussed. Some excellent products are now available that combine all these things and if you want to discuss your individual needs I suggest you call the Hormonal Advisory Service in Sydney on (02) 4653 1445 or (02) 9387 8111.

FOODS CONTAINING PLANT HORMONES

A number of different foods are sources of natural plant oestrogens and can be very helpful for **menopause** or women with **hormonal disorders** such as endometriosis, premenstrual syndrome, infertility and heavy painful periods.

These are: alfalfa, aniseed, apples, brewers yeast, barley, beetroot, cabbage, carrots, cherries, chickpeas, clover, corn, cucumber, fennel, fruit, linseeds (flaxseeds), garlic, green beans, green squash, hops, oats, olive oil, olives, papaya, parsley, peas, plums, potatoes, pumpkin, legumes (beans, peas, lentils, chickpeas), cereals, red clover, rhubarb, rice, rye, sesame seeds, soya beans, soya bean sprouts, split peas, sunflower seeds, many nuts, squash, wheat, yams.

Breast and colon cancers, heart disease, menopausal symptoms and osteoporosis have a lower incidence in Asian countries. These populations have a diet much higher in phytoestrogens than do Australians, North Americans and Europeans and it appears that plant hormones have beneficial effects not only upon the hormonal system, but also upon the immune system.

TESTIMONIALS FROM WOMEN WHO HAVE TRIED PHYTOESTROGENS

AUDREY, FROM ADELAIDE, SOUTH AUSTRALIA

I started taking phytoestrogens in powder form, combined with vitamins and minerals one year ago because of severe menopausal symptoms. I had no libido and was suffering from hot flushes and poor sleep. I had a hysterectomy when I was thirty-eight and the doctor told me that this had probably caused me to start menopause. After the hysterectomy I was alarmed to find that my hair started falling out and I had new aches and pains all over. I tried some oestrogen patches which helped the hot flushes but did not relieve my other problems. So I then consulted with a doctor who believed in natural alternatives and she prescribed a combination of herbs and foods containing phytoestrogens along with vitamin C, vitamin E, vitamin D and K and folic acid. After three months I felt my old self returning and, best of all, my hair started to thicken. I now have a good libido and it is so nice to feel like a woman again.

LORNA, FROM BOONAH, QUEENSLAND

I first became aware of phytoestrogens when viewing a segment on television. I am aged fifty-seven and have been experiencing menopausal symptoms since the age of fifty-three. As I have a strong family history of breast cancer I felt reluctant to take strong or artificial hormone replacement therapy. I decided to suffer in silence, and suffer I did, that is, until I started taking the 'magical' phtyoestrogens combined with linseed, soy, alfalfa and vitamins in powder form. Within a very short period my hot flushes diminished and what I used to call my 'fuzzy head' and vagueness disappeared, my energy levels soared and my headaches gradually stopped. I now find my disposition is much calmer and I don't suffer from moodiness nearly as much as before. My partner is delighted with the 'new' me. He did put up with a lot for too long. It is not my intention to sound like a TV commercial but I am just so relieved to feel normal again. I wanted to share this positive experience with other women who may be suffering as I did. If you are, phtyoestrogens are truly magical. I have recommended them to several women friends who are thankful for their increased well-being since beginning phtyoestrogens.

CONSTANCE, FROM ADELAIDE, SOUTH AUSTRALIA

I am definitely a naturalist and my experience of menopause has further confirmed this for me. I went through menopause last year and did not have hot flushes or anything obvious; however, my weight started to creep up and I felt very sluggish. My doctor found that my oestrogen levels were very low and that my thyroid gland was slightly underactive. I was started on hormone tablets and these did nothing at all except make me put on more weight around my stomach area. I felt bloated and ugly. I had a bone-density test and this was very good, showing that I was not at risk for osteoporosis. So I decided that these strong hormone tablets were not for me and that I would try the new phytoestrogen powder that everyone was talking about. I was already eating soy and linseed bread but this was not enough. So I decided to see a naturopath who prescribed a formula of a mixture of herbs, vitamins and foods that contain phytoestrogens in powder form. At first I did not notice much difference but then slowly over six to seven weeks I began to lose weight and feel like exercising again. My skin and hair improved and I started to look and feel more feminine. My partner said that I am definitely a natural woman and he wants me to stay that way!

HUMAN GROWTH HORMONE

The United States National Institute on Ageing is funding studies to confirm earlier findings that human growth hormone and other hormones such as the adrenal hormone DHEA and natural sex hormones (oestrogen, progesterone, testosterone) can slow and possibly reverse changes associated with ageing. The levels of these hormones drop greatly with advancing years.

Human growth hormone (HGH), produced by the pituitary gland, drops sharply with age and falls by more than 50 per cent from the peak during puberty and reaches 'older levels' by the age of forty.

Research into HGH was restricted up until the 1980s because of the inability of scientists to synthesise the complicated hormone made up of 191 amino acids. The scientific breakthrough of DNA recombinant technology in the early 1980s finally enabled HGH to be made safely in large quantities. This type of HGH is identical to the one produced by the human pituitary gland. The FDA in the USA approved the use of this type of HGH for experimental use in healthy humans in the late 1980s. An American scientist, Dr Daniel Rudman MD, at the Medical College of Wisconsin in Milwaukee, started a double-blind clinical trial using twelve healthy elderly men, aged sixty-one to eighty-one, who were given HGH three times a week for six months to restore their levels to the youthful range. By comparison with the patients who received the placebo (inactive treatment) the patients treated with HGH showed improvements that were equivalent to reversing the changes incurred during ten to twenty years of ageing. His exciting findings were published in the highly regarded *New England Journal of Medicine,* July 1990.

After this, researchers from all over the world began studying the effects of replacing growth hormone in elderly persons and the results are impressive. Additional advantageous effects shown were that HGH increases bone mass in osteoporosis, reverses the declining cardiac and lung function, improves the immune system, increases lean muscle mass, decreases the percentage of body fat, increases the capacity for exercise, increases vitality and improves sleeping. Scandinavian researchers eliminated the side effect of fluid retention found in the Rudman study by changing Rudman's three weekly HGH injections to twice daily injections of smaller doses.

Between the years 1990–92 hundreds of research studies were done on HGH's effect upon ageing and well-being. Overall conclusions were that HGH replacement therapy can be safe with proper doses and administration.

This is a breakthrough for older people of both sexes with medical problems related to ageing that could be partially reversed with HGH. Medical researchers at Stanford University summarised in 1992 the outcome of the various HGH studies by stating 'It is possible that physiologic HGH replacement therapy might REVERSE or prevent some of the inevitable sequelae of ageing.' (Reference 19)

It is important that doses are carefully controlled by a doctor who is an expert in this field. Some atheletes have abused HGH in large overdoses, which led to a condition called acromegaly which is the overgrowth of various bodily parts. Dr Eve VanCauter from the University of Chicago Medical Centre says 'All of these ideas about treating people with HGH have been directed toward people sixty-five and older. If you look at the research, people have so called 'elderly' levels by age forty. Perhaps we should be giving HGH replacement therapy earlier, rather than attempting to treat tissues that have seen little or no growth hormone for decades.'

CHAPTER FIVE

NUTRITIONAL FATIGUE

What you eat is far more important than how much you eat and I am going to give you a list of high-energy foods. The key is to 'listen' to your body, as you have different needs depending upon stress levels, exercise patterns and your body weight. You don't have to eat three large meals per day and if you don't feel hungry don't force yourself to eat a large meal; have a high-energy snack instead, such as a raw juice and dried fruit and raw nuts.

If you overload your liver with too many saturated or processed fats you will feel tired, as the liver has to break down everything you eat. The liver is the cleansing filter of your bloodstream and works very hard to remove toxic substances and waste products. So, you should strive for a diet that is low in artificial chemicals and insecticides. Try to find a source of organic produce close to where you live and you may find the local health food store has some good contacts. Chemical overload can make you feel chronically fatigued because the liver will be working overtime to break down and eliminate these toxic substances. Avoid artificial sugars as these will create unstable blood sugar levels and stress the liver further, which will not help you to lose weight.

A good liver tonic powder or capsules can help the liver to perform its many functions more efficiently and can aid with weight loss in those with a 'fatty liver'. A good liver tonic should contain the liver herbs dandelion, St Mary's thistle, globe artichoke and the amino acid taurine (see page 111).

HIGH-ENERGY FOODS

1. Raw fresh fruit and vegetables of all varieties
2. Cooked vegetables
3. Raw nuts and seeds and cold-pressed seed and vegetable oils
4. Spirulina
5. Seafood
6. Eggs (never fried)
7. Unprocessed grain foods and cereals, such as rolled oats and oat bran, barley, rye, buckwheat, wholemeal bread and rolls, wholemeal flour, rice, fresh wheatgerm
8. Dried fruit
9. Legumes (beans, peas, lentils)
10. Chicken (preferably free-range)
11. Lean fresh meat (this is optional, as you do not have to eat red meat to be healthy).

Many people think that a high-energy diet should be low in fat. This is far too simplistic because the body requires the right types of fats to produce energy.

ESSENTIAL FATTY ACIDS

The good fats are called **essential fatty acids** and are found in fish, fish oil, avocados, butternuts, corn oil, legumes, seed oils, raw nuts, raw seeds, olives, cold-pressed olive oil, evening primrose oil, flaxseed oil, sunflower seed oil, safflower seed oil, mustard seed oil, grapeseed oil, canola oil, seaweed, tofu, wheatgerm oil.

Please ensure that all your oils are **cold-pressed, very fresh** and stored in **sealed containers in the refrigerator,** otherwise these oils and the foods that contain them may become damaged (oxidised) by light, heat and air and then they are no longer beneficial.

Essential fatty acids are good for the brain, hormonal system, nervous system and liver and if you are lacking in these vital nutrients you will feel tired, moody and have a sluggish metabolism. This will make it harder for you to lose weight.

LSA—SUPER ENERGY FOOD

One delicious way to boost your intake of essential fatty acids is by grinding a mixture of **L**inseeds (flaxseeds), **S**unflower seeds and **A**lmonds. I call this powder LSA. Use three cups of linseeds, two cups of sunflower seeds and one cup of almonds and pass through a coffee grinder or food processor grinder to give a fine powder. Keep this powder in a dark glass jar in the freezer and every day take what you need from this frozen supply. It does not go hard in the freezer and this way stays fresh forever. It has a nice sweet nutty flavour. Sprinkle it on your breakfast, soups, toast and honey or add it to high-energy drinks. Even children will like this LSA mixture. It contains essential fatty acids, minerals, vitamins, fibre and plant hormones which makes it a super-energy food with anti-ageing properties.

FOR A QUICK ENERGY BOOST, EITHER AS A SNACK OR A MEAL REPLACEMENT, YOU CAN TRY AN 'ENERGY SHAKE'. TO MAKE THIS SHAKE, PLACE IN A BLENDER:

2 cups milk (skim, soy, oat or rice)
1 banana or 1 cup other chopped fresh fruit
1 tablespoon of honey
2 tablespoons of LSA

Put all the ingredients in a blender and whip it up

For variety and more calories you may add one or two raw eggs, three tablespoons of Vitari ice cream or one teaspoon of vanilla essence. I particularly enjoy using different fruit in my breakfast shake and the addition of two passionfruit makes the shake taste exquisite. There is an infinite variety of these high-energy shakes so let your creative streak run wild! Because they are light and easy to digest. they do not make you feel heavy in the stomach and they give you instant energy.

Another energy drink that I often use myself is the raw juice cocktail. Pass through the juice-extracting machine raw carrots, spinach, beetroot, apple and beet greens. Stir into this juice 1–2 teaspoons of selenium powder (see page 125) and two teaspoons of spirulina powder and mix thoroughly. This is very potent and not only will it make you feel positively dangerous, it will improve your hair and skin appearance.

HERE ARE SOME YUMMY RECIPES FOR ENERGY DRINKS

SPIRULINA HIT

1 cup apple juice
1 cup water
1 kiwi fruit, peeled and chopped
1 medium ripe banana, peeled and chopped
1 tamarillo, peeled and chopped
2 teaspoons spirulina powder

Blend all the ingredients in a blender until smooth and drink immediately.

BANANA HONEY HYPE

1 cup milk (skim, soy, oat or rice)
1 ripe banana
5 drops vanilla essence
1 teaspoon honey
1 tablespoon LSA (page 72)
1 teaspoon dessicated coconut

Blend all the ingredients in a blender and drink immediately. On a hot day, add some ice cubes.

PEAR AND APPLE ENERGISER DRINK

1 ripe pear, do not peel but remove stem
1 granny smith apple, do not peel
1 cup milk (skim, soy, oat or rice)
1 teaspoon honey
1 teaspoon LSA (page 72)
1 small scoop Vitari ice cream, optional

Place all the ingredients in blender and blend until smooth. Top with a sprinkle of cinnamon and drink immediately.

APRICOT WHIRL

5 fresh or 10 dried apricots
1/3 cup flaked almonds
2/3 cup water
2/3 cup milk (skim, soy, oat or rice)
5 drops vanilla essence
1 tablespoon honey

Blend all the ingredients in a blender until smooth and drink immediately.

FOURTEEN-DAY ENERGY DIET PLAN

I am now going to give you a **fourteen-day high-energy diet plan** to follow. This is a general guide to how you should be eating for maximum energy.

WEEK 1

MONDAY

BREAKFAST

Oat and Pear Porridge

Serves 4

1 cup rolled oats
pinch of sea salt or macrobiotic salt
4 cups water
4 medium pears peeled and chopped
1 teaspoon vanilla essence, optional
1 teaspoon honey, optional

Combine the oats, salt and half the water in a large pan; cook, stirring, for 2 minutes. Add the remaining ingredients, stirring constantly until mixture boils. Simmer, uncovered, for about 7 minutes or until soft and thickened, stirring occasionally. Serve immediately.

Also have a glass of freshly made juice of raw carrot, celery and apple.

LUNCH

Vegetable soup and fresh salad with avocado
or ***wholegrain roll or bread with salmon, tuna or sardines and fresh salad***
or ***chicken sandwich on wholegrain bread with lots of fresh salad***
or ***wholemeal pasta with tomato and/or marinara sauce, vegetables and fresh salad***
or ***grilled fish and vegetables and fresh garden salad.***

DINNER

Fish Kebabs

Serves 6

1/3 cup virgin cold-pressed olive oil
2 tablespoons lemon juice
1/2 garlic clove, crushed
1/2 teaspoon dried basil
1/2 teaspoon sea salt or macrobiotic salt
1/8 teaspoon cayenne pepper
1 kg gemfish or ling steaks, cut into 2.5 cm cubes
12 cherry tomatoes
12 button mushrooms
2–3 zucchini, cut into 12 cubes
12 lemon wedges to garnish

Combine the oil, lemon juice, garlic and seasonings. Add the fish, cover and marinate for 1 hour. Thread the fish cubes and remaining ingredients alternately on to skewers. Grill for 10–15 minutes turning frequently. Garnish with lemon wedges and serve with steamed rice and fresh garden salad.

TUESDAY

BREAKFAST

2 boiled or poached eggs with wholemeal or rye toast
2 pieces of fresh fruit

LUNCH

Same as Monday, take your choice.

DINNER

Penne and Vegetables with Feta Cheese

Serves 6-8

1 onion, chopped
1/3 cup virgin cold-pressed olive oil
3 medium carrots, sliced diagonally
1 cup broccoli florets
2 cups vegetable stock
1/2 cup white wine
2 tablespoons tomato paste
1/2 teaspoon freshly ground black pepper
800 g can tomatoes, drained and chopped
170 g jar artichokes hearts, drained
1 tablespoon finely chopped basil
1 tablespoon finely chopped parsley
1 tablespoon finely chopped thyme
6 cups penne pasta, uncooked
1/2 cup crumbled feta cheese

Sauté the onion gently in oil for 3 minutes. Add the carrots and broccoli, vegetable stock, wine, tomato paste and pepper and simmer uncovered for 5 minutes. Add the tomatoes, artichoke hearts, basil, parsley and thyme to the mixture and simmer for further 5-10 minutes. Meanwhile, cook the pasta in lots of boilng water until just tender, drain. Place the pasta and vegetables into a large bowl, pour in the mixed vegetables and toss. Sprinkle the feta cheese on top and serve immediately.

WEDNESDAY

BREAKFAST

Pancakes

These pancakes are best made just before serving.

Serves 4

2 cups rolled oats
2 cups soy or oat milk
1/3 cup (90 ml) maple syrup or rice malt syrup
4 x 60 g free-range eggs, lightly beaten
1/4 cup orange juice
1 1/2 cups oat bran
1 tablespoon self-raising flour
1/2 teaspoon sea salt or macrobiotic salt

Combine the oats and the milk in large bowl. Stand for 10 minutes. Stir in the remaining ingredients. Pour 1/3 cup of the mixture into a non-stick pan which has been lightly coated with cold-pressed oil. Cook until browned on both sides. Repeat with the remaining mixture. Serve with fresh fruit (e.g. strawberries, banana, kiwifrut, etc.) or squeezed lemon, orange or grapefruit juice and honey on top. Sprinkle with LSA (see page 72) You may add some Vitari ice cream on top.

LUNCH

Same as Monday, take your choice.

DINNER

Baked Fuity Chicken

Serves 4

1/4 cup wholemeal flour
1 teaspoon sea salt or macrobiotic salt
pepper, to taste
1.5 kg chicken pieces
1/3 cup virgin cold-pressed olive oil
2 cups fresh orange juice
juice of 1 lemon
2 cups mixed dried fruit
1/4 cup brown sugar

Preheat the oven to 180°C. Place the flour, salt and pepper in a plastic bag. Add the chicken pieces and toss until completely covered. Sauté the chicken in the hot oil until brown, remove from the pan and place in an ovenproof dish. Place the remaining ingredients into the pan and stir until boiling. Pour the fruit sauce mixture over the chicken, cover and bake in the oven for 1 hour.

THURSDAY

BREAKFAST

Homemade Muesli

This recipe makes a large quantity; store in an airtight container in the refrigerator.

2 cups whole oats
3 cups rolled oats
1½ cups oat or rice bran
1 cup sunflower seed kernels
¾ cup pepitas (pumpkin seed kernels)
¾ cup cashews, chopped
½ cup slivered almonds
½ cup sesame seeds
½ cup sunflower seeds
½ cup shredded coconut
½ cup virgin cold-pressed olive oil
½ cup honey
1 teaspoon vanilla essence
½ cup raisins, chopped
½ cup seeded prunes, chopped
½ cup dried apricots, sliced
½ cup seeded dates, sliced

Place the whole oats in large heatproof bowl. Cover well with boiling water, cover and stand overnight. Drain, rinse well and pat dry. Combine the whole oats with the remaining dry ingredients, except the fruit, in a large baking dish; mix well. Bake uncovered in a moderate oven for about 40 minutes or until lightly browned, stirring occasionally. Let cool, add dried fruit then serve with soy or oat milk. The mixture must be stored in the refrigerator and is suitable for freezing. If you prefer, you may skip the baking step, just mix only the dry ingredients together and eat this muesli raw.

LUNCH

Same as Monday, take your choice.

DINNER

Orange Roughy with Fruit and Honey

Serves 3–5

6 orange roughy or bream fillets
½ cup virgin cold-pressed olive oil
garlic powder, to taste
black pepper, to taste
2 green apples, sliced 1 cm thick
juice of 1 lemon
honey, to taste

Preheat the grill to a low heat. Tear six 30 cm-long pieces of alumimium foil and lightly oil. Place one fillet of fish in the centre of each piece of foil. Top each fillet with ½ teaspoon of oil, some garlic powder, black pepper, ⅙ of the apple slices and lemon juice, drizzle with honey to taste. Wrap the foil tightly around the fillets. Place the foil parcels under the grill and cook for 20–25 minutes, turning once. Serve with steamed brown rice.

F R I D A Y

BREAKFAST

Rushers Shake

Makes 2 cups

1½ cups vanilla or plain soy or oat milk
½ cup crushed ice
1 banana
6 strawberries
1–2 passionfruit
3 tablespoons LSA (page 72)
3 tablespoons Vitari ice cream or 1 tablespoon honey
2 x 60 g raw eggs, optional

Blend together and serve immediately.

LUNCH

Same as Monday, take your choice.

DINNER

Tofu, Vegetable and Cashew Stir-Fry

Best made close to serving.

Serves 4

¼ cup virgin cold-pressed olive oil
250 g firm tofu
1 medium onion, finely chopped
1 medium green capsicum, chopped
1 teaspoon freshly grated ginger
1 stick celery, chopped
2 medium carrots, sliced
1 cup shredded cabbage
8 button mushrooms, sliced
¾ cup cashew nuts
1 cup vegetable stock
soy sauce, to taste

Heat the oil in a wok or frying pan, add the tofu and cook until lightly browned, remove with a slotted spoon. Add the onion, capsicum, ginger, celery and carrots and stir-fry until softened. Add the cabbage, mushrooms and cashew nuts, stir-fry until softened. Return the tofu to the wok with the stock, cover and simmer until the vegetables are soft. Stir in the soy sauce. Serve with steamed brown rice and salad.

SATURDAY

BREAKFAST

Scrambled Tofu and Vegetables
Serves 4

2 teaspoons dark sesame oil
1 small onion, chopped
1 small carrot, chopped
1 stick celery, finely chopped
1 teaspoon freshly grated ginger
300 g firm tofu, crumbled
1 tablespoon fresh coriander leaves, chopped
1/4 teaspoon ground turmeric
1/4 teaspoon ground black pepper
2 teaspoons tamari or shoyu
4 slices sourdough bread, toasted
2 teaspoons sesame seeds, toasted

Heat the sesame oil gently in a large frying pan, add the onion, carrot and celery and cook, stirring, until onion is soft. Add the ginger, crumbled tofu, coriander, turmeric, pepper and tamari. Simmer, covered, for 3 minutes or until vegetables are tender. Serve on the toasted sourdough bread, and sprinkle with the sesame seeds.

LUNCH

Same as Monday, take your choice.

DINNER

Spicy Chicken with Peanuts
Serves 3–4
1 tablespoon cornflour
1 tablespoon low-salt soy sauce
1 egg white
1 garlic clove, crushed
500 g skinless chicken breasts, diced
3 tablespoons virgin cold-pressed olive oil
1/3 cup raw, fresh unsalted peanuts
1/4 teaspoon cayenne pepper
1 large green capsicum, seeded and cut into fine strips
warm flour tortillas
Sauce
1 teaspoon cornflour
1/4 teaspoon ground ginger
1 teaspoon dry sherry
2 tablespoons low-salt soy sauce
2 teaspoons honey
2 teaspoons red wine vinegar

Blend the cornflour, soy sauce, egg white and garlic. Add the chicken and mix well. Cover and chill for 30 minutes. In a large frying pan, heat 2 tablespoons of the oil, add the peanuts and cayenne pepper. Fry until the peanuts are brown. Remove peanuts with a slotted spoon then drain on paper towels. Add the remaining oil to the pan, heat and stir-fry the drained chicken for 2 minutes. Add the capsicum and cook a further 2 minutes.

Blend the sauce ingredients together well and add to the pan, stirring until boiling. Mix in the peanuts.

Pass the tortillas and the chicken filling around so that everyone may fill their own tortillas. Roll the tortilla to enclose the filling and eat with fingers.

Serve with a fresh garden salad.

SUNDAY

BREAKFAST

Jaffles

Suggested fillings are baked beans, cooked mushrooms, free-range eggs. Serve with some fresh salad or vegetables on the side.

Heat the jaffle iron and brush lightly with cold-pressed oil. Place wholemeal or rye bread into the jaffle iron and fill with one of the suggested fillings. Close and cook for 4–6 minutes until brown and crisp.

LUNCH

Same as Monday, take your choice.

DINNER

Vegetarian Spaghetti Neopolitan

1 cup green lentils, cooked, in plenty of water for about 45 minutes
2 onions, peeled and sliced
2 tablespoons virgin cold-pressed olive oil
1–2 garlic cloves, minced
1 large carrot, diced
3 tablespoons canned chopped tomatoes or tomato purée
1 tablespoon chopped fresh basil
sea salt or macrobiotic salt and black pepper to taste
(If you want to be naughty, add a slosh of red wine!)

wholemeal spaghetti (remember it takes longer to cook than white but be sure it is 'al dente.')

Drain the lentils, but save the liquid. Sauté the onion in oil for about 5 minutes to brown lightly, then add the garlic and carrot and 1 cup of lentil water. Cover the saucepan and simmer gently for 10 minutes or until the vegetables are tender. Stir in the tomatoes, basil, lentils and enough of the saved lentil water to give a thick moist consistency. Add salt.

Be sure to begin cooking the spaghetti about 10 minutes before the sauce will be finished. Drain the spaghetti well, return to warm pan and toss with black pepper. Serve the sauce piping hot, poured over the spaghetti in a warmed bowl. Serve with a fresh leafy salad.

If you feel like some seafood with this, sauté, in a small amount of cold-pressed oil, a selection of mixed seafood such as prawns, mussels, calamari, octopus, etc.

SUNDAY

IF YOU FEEL LIKE A MEAT DISH TONIGHT, TRY THIS ONE:

Ginger Lamb Stir-Fry
Serves 4

375 g lean boneless lamb, all fat removed and cut into thin strips
2 teaspoons dry sherry
1 tablespoon low-salt soy sauce
½ teaspoon sesame oil
2 teaspoons olive oil
1 medium leek, cut into 6 cm long strips
1 shallot, chopped
2 garlic cloves, thinly sliced
2 teaspoons freshly grated ginger

Place the lamb in a shallow dish. Combine the sherry, soy sauce and sesame oil and pour over the lamb; refrigerate for 30 minutes. Heat the olive oil in a wok or frying pan, add the undrained lamb in batches, stir-frying until just tender; remove. Add the leek strips, stir-fry the shallot, garlic and ginger, 2 minutes. Return the lamb and marinade liquid to the wok, stir-fry until cooked. Serve with 3–4 cooked vegetables and a fresh garden salad. You may also have some brown rice or pasta if your appetite is large.

WEEK 2

MONDAY

BREAKFAST

Fruit compote sprinkled with toasted muesli.

Exotic compotes can be made from dried fruits. They are always in season and it saves chopping more fresh fruit than is required. The choice is yours!

Place the selected dried fruits (about half a kilo if you want to store some) in a shallow pan with water and simmer slowly until the fruit is tender. Serve with toasted muesli, granola, LSA (page 72), or soy yoghurt.

LUNCH

1. Some yummy sandwich ideas:

Try some rye, multigrain loaf or sour dough bread. Use pita bread if you want a lot of filling.

Spread your choice of bread with avocado and/or brazil nut spread or other nut spreads, then add some grated beetroot, grated carrot, alfalfa sprouts, and a little sweet onion. You may toast the sandwiches, if you desire. For a sweet filling try honey, mashed banana and cinnamon—this is delicious as an open sandwich too. Simply toast your choice of bread, add the filling on top, then place under a grill for a few minutes.

OR

2. Vegetarian Hamburger

Use wholemeal rolls rather than hamburger buns.

Makes 3–4

The burger pattie

1 cup cooked and puréed green lentils
60 g egg, lightly beaten
1 onion, chopped and sautéed (you may use garlic as well)
1/4 cup crushed nuts (walnuts work well)
1 cup mashed potato
soy sauce, to taste
houmos spread
tomato sauce, optional
some salad vegetables

Mix all the pattie ingredients together, form into patties and flatten slightly. Lightly oil and heat a heavy pan and fry patties until brown on both sides. Spread houmos and tomato sauce on both sides of rolls then add patties. Serve with a fresh garden salad.

OR

3. Vegetable Fritters

2 cups grated vegetables of your choice
1/2 cup wholemeal self-raising flour
vegetable salt, to taste
2 x 60 g eggs, beaten

Thoroughly mix all the ingredients together. (Some vegetables have a lot of liquid, so if the mixture is too watery, add more flour.) Form the mixture into patties. Lightly oil a heavy pan and cook the patties slowly until brown on one side, then turn over and cook the other side. Serve on wholemeal rolls with tomato sauce and/or houmos.

For a special salad plate:
Sauté a sliced onion with 2 teaspoons of ground coriander and 100–150 g of drained, sliced button mushrooms. When just soft, add 1½ tablespoons of soy sauce and a can of drained butter beans or your favourite bean mix. Mix thoroughly and chill for at least 2 hours.

OR

4. Tuna Curry Stir-Fry
Serves 2 (or 1 big eater!)

1 carrot, julienned
1 stick celery, julienned
2 spring onions, cut into small lengths
½ garlic clove, crushed
2 tablespoons virgin cold-pressed olive oil
180 g can Greenseas Tuna Cuisine Tuna Curry
2 tablespoons of chopped coriander or a sprinkle of the powder

Stir-fry the vegetables and garlic in oil until tender but crisp. Add the tuna curry and coriander, cook until heated through. Serve with steamed jasmine rice.

DINNER

Lemon Chicken Stir-Fry
Serves 3–4

2 tablespoons low-salt soy sauce
1 tablespoon cornflour
1 tablespoon sherry
3 boneless half chicken breasts, cut into strips
¼ cup lemon juice
2 tablespoons rice wine vinegar
4 teaspoons honey
1 teaspoon grated lemon zest
3 tablespoons virgin cold-pressed olive oil
3 spring onions
1 carrot, sliced
1 cup sliced capsicum
1 garlic clove, minced

Mix the soy sauce, cornflour and sherry until smooth. Toss the chicken strips in the mixture until well coated. Combine the lemon juice, vinegar, honey and lemon zest in a separate bowl. Heat 1 tablespoon of the oil in a wok or large frying pan over a medium heat. Stir in the vegetables and the garlic, sauté until tender but crisp. With a slotted spoon remove the vegetables from the pan and set aside. Add the remaining oil to the pan and heat. Stir-fry the chicken with the marinade until just cooked through. Stir in the lemon mixture, reduce heat and simmer, covered, for 2 minutes, then stir in the vegetables to heat through. Serve with hot rice and a fresh garden salad.

TUESDAY

BREAKFAST

Home-made Crunchy Granola

Make up on the weekend to have it ready for an easy week day breakfast.

Toast 4 cups of rolled oats with half a cup of honey in a shallow baking dish in a warm oven. Stir often until golden. Take from the oven and stir in 1 cup of LSA (page 72), or use wheatgerm, ½ cup of chopped raw nuts, ½ cup of raisins, apricots, prunes or sultanas. Serve with soy, oat, rice or skim milk and any fresh fruit.

LUNCH

Choose anything from Monday lunches or have

Tofu Brochettes

Thread skewers alternately with cubed tofu and vegetables or an exotic fruit selection such as grapes, pineapple and mango. Coat lightly with mango chutney. Pre-heat the grill and cook for 5 minutes until very hot and just starting to brown. Serve immediately sprinkled very lightly with your favourite herb and LSA (page 72). Serve with fresh garden salad.

DINNER

Grilled fish of your choice, jacket potatoes and mixed vegetable salad

OR

Spinch, Tomato and Walnut Lasagne

Serves 6

375 g lasagne pasta
1½ cups ricotta cheese
2 x 60 g eggs
1 dessertspoon chopped parsley
½ teaspoon sea salt or macrobiotic salt
250 g packet frozen spinach, thawed
1½ cups Italian-style tomato sauce (bottled or home-made)
½ cup chopped walnuts
1 cup grated mozzarella cheese
2 tablespoons parmesan cheese

Cook lasagne according to directions on packet. Whisk together ricotta and eggs in a bowl, stir in parsley and salt. Set aside. Press out as much liquid as possible from thawed spinach. In an oiled 20 x 30 cm, shallow ovenproof dish, spread a layer of tomato sauce. Place a layer of lasagne sheets on top. Spread over a layer of spinach and a layer of ricotta cheese mixture. Sprinkle over some chopped walnuts. Repeat layers. On the top layer of lasagne, sprinkle over mozzarella and parmesan cheese. Bake in a moderate oven for 30–40 minutes. Serve with a fresh garden salad.

WEDNESDAY

BREAKFAST

Semolina Start

½ cup semolina
1½ cups of soy, oat, rice or skim milk
½ cup of dried mixed fruit
¼ cup LSA (page 72)

Mix all the ingredients together in a heavy saucepan. Heat slowly and stir carefully until soft and thickened. Serve with some soy yoghurt or honey, if desired.

LUNCH

Same as Monday, take your choice.

DINNER

Celery Plus Soup

This is nice on cold days and is not only tasty but contains anti-oxidant vegetables to help cleanse the liver and boost the immune system.

2 cups chopped celery
1 cup chopped broccoli florets
½ cup chopped parsley
1 large onion, chopped
1 large potato, chopped
½ teaspoon lemon pepper
¼ teaspoon mustard powder
sea salt or macrobiotic salt or lemon juice, to taste
soy milk

Place all the ingredients in large saucepan, barely cover with water and simmer gently until soft. Cool slightly, place in a food processor or blender and purée until smooth. Return to saucepan, add salt or lemon juice and enough soy milk to form a smooth thick soup.

FOLLOWED BY

Zucchini Slice

5 x 60 g eggs, lightly beaten
400 g zucchini, coarsely grated
1 large onion, finely chopped
2 medium carrots, coarsely grated
¼ cup virgin cold-pressed olive oil
½ cup finely chopped parsley
½ teaspoon lemon pepper
sea salt or macrobiotic salt to taste
1 tablespoon cooked soya beans, optional
1 cup wholemeal self-raising flour

Combine all the ingredients, except the flour. Mix well, then fold in the flour until blended well. Pour into a 28 x 18 cm lamington tin and bake in a moderate oven for 30–40 minutes. Serve warm with a fresh salad or rice.

This can also be cut into wedges and taken cold to a picnic.

THURSDAY

BREAKFAST

Wholemeal or rye toast with tahini or nut paste spread, sliced banana, honey and LSA (page 72). 2 pieces of fresh fruit.

LUNCH

Same as Monday, take your choice.

DINNER

Vegetarian-style Nut Roast with Apricot or Mango Stuffing

Serves 2

1 large onion, chopped
4 tomatoes, chopped
1 tablespoon virgin cold-pressed olive oil
1 cup vegetable stock or water
pinch of mixed herbs
2 cups breadcrumbs (wholemeal, if possible)
½ cup cashew nuts, chopped
½ cup brazil nuts, chopped
pinch of sea salt or macrobiotic salt
black pepper, to taste
nutmeg, to taste
60 g egg, beaten
1 teaspoon sesame seeds

Stuffing

1 cup dried apricots or mango
(cover with water and soak for 4 hours)
1 tablespoon lemon juice
1 dessertspoon virgin cold-pressed olive oil
pinch of sea salt or macrobiotic salt
½ teaspoon mixed spice
1 cup breadcrumbs
60 g egg, beaten

Sauté the onions and tomatoes in oil until soft. Add the stock, remove from the heat. In a large bowl, mix herbs, breadcrumbs, nuts, salt, pepper and nutmeg. Add tomato and onion mixture, eggs and stir well. Thoroughly oil a large tin with some cold-pressed oil and sprinkle with the sesame seeds to prevent the roast from sticking.

Spoon half the roast mixture into the prepared tin, then add stuffing. Spoon the remaining mixture on top and smooth over with a fork. Bake in a medium oven for 40–45 minutes until brown and firm to the touch. Let stand for about 10 minutes before turning out.

To make the stuffing: Simmer the apricots and/or mangoes in their soaking water for half an hour until soft. Drain and chop finely, add lemon juice, oil, salt, spice, breadcrumbs and egg. Mix thoroughly.

FRIDAY

BREAKFAST

Home-made muesli (page 79) with skim, rice, soy or oat milk and soy yoghurt with 2 pieces of fresh fruit.

LUNCH

Same as Monday, take your choice.

DINNER

Patricia's Great Standby

Make up a huge pot of thick soup and there will be some left over for weekend visitors!

8 large chicken drumsticks, skinned
½ cup red lentils
½ cup pearl barley
3 large carrots, chopped
3 celery stalks, chopped
1 head broccoli, finely chopped
2 onions, chopped
any other vegetables you desire
2 x 375 ml Campbell's All Natural Chicken Stock

Place the drumsticks in a saucepan and cover with water, simmer for about an hour. When tender, remove the drumsticks, reserving the stock, and allow to cool.

Half fill a saucepan with water, add the lentils and pearl barley and simmer for ½ an hour. Add raw vegetables and simmer gently until soft (do not overcook), topping up liquid level with reserved chicken stock when necessary.

Take a very large container—a crock pot is perfect—and pour in the vegetables with their water, if there is any left. Add the Campbell's chicken stock.

Carefully pull the flesh from the drumsticks taking great care not to include the sharp spiky little bones. Cut the meat into small pieces and add to the soup. Only reheat what you intend to eat; the remainder can be frozen. Serve with thick toast or foccacia bread, spread with houmos or nut paste spread.

When you want to use the frozen soup, you could, if you wish, add a little bottled V8 Vegetable Juice or bottled carrot juice which makes the soup very sweet.

SATURDAY

BREAKFAST

For a lazy breakfast on the weekend you could have a giant smoothie made with your selection of fresh fruit. Use soy, rice, skim or oat milk. Smoothies can have LSA or wheatgerm thrown in, as well as honey or maple syrup. See page 73 for energy shake recipes.

If you haven't got a blender then have one of the cereals mentioned on previous days, with some fresh fruit.

LUNCH

Anything from Monday or make an amazing fruit salad.

If in season, start with very ripe nectarines and tangellos. Consider also using blueberries, raspberries, sultana grapes, canned or fresh mango pieces, canned or fresh mandarin pieces. Or tinned fruit salad as a base with your own fresh section tossed in. You can even have some Vitari ice cream on the top!

DINNER

Risotto alla Ziliani

Serve with grilled sea perch

This risotto (rice) recipe can be adjusted according to whether you want more, less, or to have some left over.

1 tablespoon virgin cold-pressed olive oil
1–1½ cups unpolished brown rice, washed and drained
1–2 x 375 ml Campbell's All Natural Stock, Chicken or Vegetable
1 medium onion, finely chopped
garlic, fresh or powdered to taste
pinch of chilli powder, if desired
1 small celery stick, chopped
1 cup chopped capsicum, red and green
1 cup baby peas
5 button mushrooms, sliced
1 cup sweet corn kernels

Heat the oil gently in a large pan. Cover the base of the pan with as much rice as you want—remember it grows when it's cooking! Fry until rice browns a little, stirring constantly. Remove from heat and allow to cool just a little. Pour over 1 carton of the stock. If you have a huge amount of rice then use 2 cartons but taste before adding any salt as you probably won't need it. Return to a low heat and allow rice to soak up the stock, while you prepare the vegetables. Add the onion, garlic, chilli powder, celery and capsicum. As the stock is absorbed, add hot water. Cover and gently cook for 10 minutes, then add the peas, mushrooms and corn kernels. Top up the water level and cover. Simmer till rice is tender. The rice will take quite a while if using unpolished brown rice. If you are in a great hurry use white rice but it does not have the same nutritional value.

This dish can be eaten as a main meal or used as a side dish with grilled sea perch and is nice to eat cold for lunch the next day.

SUNDAY

BREAKFAST

Soy and linseed bread toasted and spread with either nut spread or tahini, sliced banana and LSA (see page 72). You may spread honey on the toast too, if you have a sweet tooth. Have an apple and some freshly squeezed orange juice

LUNCH

The BBQ—outside or inside

Marinated BBQ Chicken Breasts

Mix together 2 tablespoons tomato sauce, 2 tablespoons honey, 4 tablespoons soy sauce, 2 tablespoons lemon juice, ½ teaspoon grated ginger, or you may use our spicy pear savoury sauce as a marinade, if you prefer, and it is healthier. Place 500 g sliced boneless chicken breast pieces in an ovenproof dish, cover with the marinade and refrigerate. After an hour or so, turn over the chicken. These sauces work well on any type of meat but we won't eat sausages will we?!

Or make some vegetarian burgers from Soy Feast Burger Mix or other similar products.

Barbecued Vegetables

Most vegetables work well but here are a few suggestions: red and yellow capsicums, thickly sliced egg plant and sweet potato, and onions cut in half. Some people like them wrapped in foil, while others like them straight on the hot plate.

Spicy Pear Savoury Sauce

This is a delicious sauce for all cooked meats and a great marinade for barbecued meats. You may like to make this one for the chicken instead of the more conventional tomato sauce marinade. Use ½ cup per 500 g of sliced chicken.

1 kg pears, peeled, cored and diced
440 g can tomatoes
2 tablespoons honey
2 medium onions, diced
1 cup malt vinegar
½ cup chopped seeded dates
½ cup chopped seeded raisins
1 dessertspoon finely chopped ginger
1 dessertspoon mustard powder
1 teaspoon lemon pepper
2 tablespoons Worcestershire sauce
chilli powder, to taste

Place all the ingredients in a saucepan and bring slowly to the boil. Simmer for ¾ hour stirring often with a wooden spoon. If you like it hot and spicy, add ½ teaspoon of chilli powder while cooking. Cool slightly. Purée in a blender. Place in clean glass containers and seal while still warm.

The marinade for the vegetables

½ cup virgin cold-pressed olive oil
1 large garlic clove, crushed
2 tablespoons finely chopped fresh mixed summer herbs, e.g. parsely, basil, chives
vegetable salt to taste
freshly ground pepper, to taste

Combine all the marinade ingredients in a screw-top jar. Shake well. Brush the vegetables with the marinade and set aside for about ½ hour. Before cooking, brush the vegetables once more with the marinade and sprinkle with some extra seasoning.

You may barbecue these over a grill, turning frequently OR pierce each vegetable with a fork, place on a sheet of foil, pour over some marinade, wrap and cook, on the hotplate, occasionally turning until soft.

Serve with a fresh salad of lettuce, cherry tomatoes, alfalfa sprouts and a dressing of virgin cold-pressed olive oil and balsamic vinegar. Sprinkle lightly with basil.

You may also make a potato salad with onion and sliced hard-boiled eggs covered with a light mayonnaise.

Nice healthy dips for the barbecue

These dips are great with healthy crackers, such as rice cakes, Ryvitas, Vita-Weat biscuits, etc. Try cutting pita bread into small strips and bake in a slow oven until dry and crisp. This pita bread keeps well in an airtight jar for a few weeks and is always ready for unexpected guests. You may also use vegetable sticks if you wish.

Garlic Dip

6 large garlic cloves (use more if you love it strong!) crushed and pounded with ½ teaspoon sea salt or macrobiotic salt until smooth. Add 2 cups of mashed potato, ½ cup of cold-pressed olive oil and 2 tablespoons of lemon juice. Mix until well combined. If you enjoy a real healthy zing, add 1 teaspoon of finely chopped chilli. Cover and let it stand for at least 1 hour for the best flavour.

Quick Salmon Dip or Spread

170 g can pink salmon, drained
1 dessertspoon ricotta cheese or soy yoghurt
1 tablespoon chopped parsley
1 tablespoon chopped spring onions
1 dessertspoon lemon juice
black pepper, to taste

Mash salmon (including bones) and add all the other ingredients. Mix until well combined and smooth.

Handy hint for dips

If ever dips are too thin, add a small amount of wholemeal flour, LSA (page 72) or wheatgerm until thick enough. This gives a nice nutty flavour.

Dessert can be any of the delights from the Sweet Treats section of this book (pages 94–102).

DINNER

Fast Tasty Pasta

375 g wholemeal pasta shells
$1\frac{1}{2}$ cups each broccoli and cauliflower, finely chopped
$1\frac{1}{2}$ cups soy or oat milk
200 g ricotta cheese
1 cup chopped parsley
$\frac{1}{2}$ cup finely chopped shallots or onion
$\frac{1}{2}$ teaspoon lemon pepper
sea salt or macrobiotic salt, to taste
420 g can pink salmon, drained and flaked

Cook the pasta in large pot of boiling water for 8 minutes. Add the broccoli and cauliflower and cook for another 3–4 minutes. Drain and place in large bowl. Meanwhile, warm the milk and blend in the ricotta, the parsley, onion and pepper and salt. Pour over the drained pasta and mix through salmon. Place in a lightly oiled casserole dish, cover and bake at 180°C for 15 minutes. Serve with a fresh green salad and crusty bread (no butter or margarine).

NATURAL SWEET TREATS

These sweet treats will not sap your energy. They are made with natural ingredients and provided you do not have large servings and do not over indulge, you will find them yummy additions to the energy diet. We are all human and our taste buds crave something sweet when we feel a little bored or naughty. Our sweet recipes do not contain artificial sweeteners as these will cause low blood sugar levels, fatigue and excessive hunger. If you suffer with hypoglycaemia or candida you will need to watch your consumption of sweets because excessive amounts will make these conditions much worse.

These sweet treats were designed by the one and only Audrey Tea who is a long time friend of mine. They have been tried and tested in the kitchen of Audrey Tea and eaten by thousands of her willing subjects. We are indeed lucky to have these recipes because she is a fabulous cook. Audrey Tea is my recipe tester and often makes me samples of her yummy recipes. Her famous recipes have been enjoyed by people everywhere. I would like to share them with you. They come with sunshine and laughter just like Audrey Tea herself!

Pear Petit Fours

1 cup chopped dried pears
½ cup chopped dried apricots
½ cup chopped cashews
½ cup shredded coconut
1 tablespoon lemon juice
1 tablespoon honey
400 g can coconut cream
extra cashews, for decoration

Mix all the ingredients together with enough coconut cream to bind the mixture together. Stand, covered, for 1 hour. If the mixture is too dry, add a little more coconut cream to hold it together. Roll into small balls, press a cashew nut into the top of each and place in small confectionery paper patty cups. Cover and store in the refrigerator. These last for days and are nice for morning or afternoon tea.

Pear Truffles

1 cup dried pears, minced or finely chopped
¾ cup seeded raisins, minced or finely chopped
1 teaspoon preserved ginger, minced or finely chopped
1 tablespoon honey
1 tablespoon LSA (page 72)
1 cup toasted coconut

Combine the pears, raisins and ginger with the honey and LSA and ½ of the coconut. Mix well. Form mixture into small balls and roll in the remaining coconut. Slightly flatten to form thick patties. Refrigerate until firm, then store in the fridge in an airtight container.

Apple Muffins

Can be made a day ahead

Makes 12 muffins

3 tablespoons cold-pressed almond oil
1½ cups wholemeal self-raising flour
½ teaspoon mixed spice
½ teaspoon ground cinnamon
½ cup sultanas
2 x 60 g eggs, lightly beaten
1 cup chopped unsweetened cooked apple or canned pie apple
1 tablespoon honey
½ cup skim, oat or soy milk

Coat a 12-hole muffin pan with 1 tablespoon of almond oil or use paper muffin cups. Sift the dry ingredients into a large bowl and stir in the sultanas. Add the eggs, remaining oil, apple, honey and milk; stir with large spoon until just combined. Spoon the mixture into the prepared pan, then bake in a moderate oven for about 20 minutes.

Banana Cake

1 cup (approximately 2 large) over-ripe bananas, mashed
1 cup wholemeal self-raising flour
¾ cup rolled oat flakes
pinch of sea salt or macrobiotic salt
⅔ cup chopped raisins
½ cup chopped walnuts
⅓ cup cold-pressed sunflower oil
2 x 60 g eggs, lightly beaten
½ teaspoon bicarbonate of soda
1 teaspoon vanilla essence

Brush the base and sides of a 14 x 21 cm loaf pan with extra cold-pressed oil. Combine all the ingredients in large bowl and mix until the consistency is soft and moist. Spread the mixture into the prepared pan. Bake in a moderate oven for about 50 minutes. Let stand for about 15 minutes before turning the cake onto a wire rack to cool.

Fruit and Nut Energy Bars

1½ cups wholemeal self-raising flour
¼ cup raw brown sugar
1 cup chopped dates
1 cup chopped walnuts
½ cup virgin cold-pressed olive oil
2 tablespoons golden syrup or honey

Mix the flour and all the other dry ingredients together in a large bowl. Put oil and golden syrup or honey into a saucepan and stir over a low heat until melted and combined. Cool, then mix into the dry ingredients. Place mixture into an oiled, greaseproof paper lined 22 cm square cake tin and bake in a moderate oven for about 1/2 hour or until golden brown. While still warm, cut into bars with a sharp knife. Store in an airtight container.

Fruit Chews

1 cup nut paste (almond, macadamia or hazelnut)
1/2 cup honey
1/4 cup raw sugar
3 cups Rice Bubbles
1 teaspoon vanilla essence
1/2 cup sultanas
1/2 cup currants

Combine the nut paste, honey and sugar in large saucepan. Stir over a low heat until the mixture is dissolved. Add the remaining ingredients and mix until everything is well coated. Press firmly into an oiled, greasproof paper lined 28 x 18 cm lamington tin. Refrigerate for 1 hour, cut into fingers.

Reward Treat Banana Cake

1/2 cup cold-pressed oil
1/2 cup raw sugar
2 x 60 g eggs
2 large ripe bananas, mashed
3 tablespoons soy or skim milk
1 level teaspoon bicarbonate of soda
1 teaspoon vanilla essence
2 cups self-raising flour (half white/half wholemeal), sifted
1 teaspoon cinnamon, optional
chopped walnuts, optional

Beat the oil and sugar until smooth, add the eggs, beat well, then add the mashed banana. Mix the soy milk, bicarbonate of soda and vanilla essence together and add alternately with sifted flour until all ingredients are folded smoothly together. Place mixture in an oiled and greaseproof paper lined 23 cm tin. Sprinkle with cinnamon and/or chopped walnuts, if desired. Cook in a moderate oven for about 45 minutes or until a skewer comes out clean. Cool in the tin for about 10 minutes before turning out onto a wire cake rack.

MORNING OR AFTERNOON TEA TREATS

Audrey's Health Hints

Many loaf and bar cakes are served with butter or margarine. To avoid this extra fat, try a thin spread of honey, tahini, fruit jam or nut spread (macadamia, hazelnut, brazil or almond).

Any recipe that has a bran-type cereal content can have delicious added flavour if you substitute the same amount of LSA mixture (page 72) for the bran-type cereal.

To remove tea and coffee stains from mugs and cups, mix a little bicarbonate of soda with lemon juice and apply with a clean cloth, then rinse in water.

Grainy Apricot Loaf

1 cup rice bran
3/4 cup brown sugar
125 g dried apricots, chopped
2 tablespoons honey
1 cup soy, rice or skim milk
1 cup wholemeal self-raising flour, sifted

Combine the rice bran, sugar, apricots, honey and milk and mix well. Let the mixture stand for about 2 hours in refrigerator. Fold in the flour and mix well. Line a 23 x 12 cm loaf tin and oil the base and sides with cold-pressed oil. Put the mixture into the loaf tin, then bake in a moderate oven for 1 hour or until a skewer comes out clean. Cool, slice and serve.

Tangy Fruit Loaf

1/4 cup cold-pressed oil
1/2 cup brown sugar
60 g egg
3 sliced bananas
1/2 cup chopped dates
juice of 1 lemon
1/2 cup chopped pecan or walnuts
1 1/2 cups wholemeal self-raising flour, sifted
1/2 cup wheatgerm
1/2 teaspoon bicarbonate of soda

Heat the oil and sugar in a saucepan stirring until dissolved. Cool. Add the egg and beat well. Stir in the bananas, dates, lemon juice and nuts. Add the flour, wheatgerm and bicarbonate of soda. Fold in and blend well. Pour into an oiled 23 x 12 cm loaf tin and bake in a moderate oven for about 1 hour.

Spicy Apple Fruit Cake

60 g egg
1 cup brown sugar
1/2 cup cold-pressed oil
1/4 cup sweet sherry
500 g mixed dried fruit
3 apples, peeled and grated
1/2 cup chopped walnuts
2 cups wholemeal self-raising flour, sifted
2 teaspoons bicarbonate of soda
1/2 teaspoon each of nutmeg, mixed spice, ginger and cinnamon

Beat together the egg and the sugar. Add the oil and sherry and mix well. Add the dried fruit, apples and nuts and combine well. Add the flour, bicarbonate of soda and spices and mix until well combined. Place the mixture in a large loaf or 20 cm-square oiled and lined tin and bake for about 1 hour in a moderate oven. The cake is ready when a skewer comes out clean.

No Eggs Raisin Nut Loaf

1/4 cup cold-pressed oil
1 cup brown sugar
1 cup water
1 tablespoon honey
250 g chopped raisins
2 teaspoons mixed spice
1 cup white plain flour, sifted
1 cup wholemeal self-raising flour, sifted
1 teaspoon bicarbonate of soda
1/2 cup chopped pecans or walnuts (or both)

Place the oil, sugar, water, honey, raisins and spice into a large saucepan over a medium heat. Stir until the mixture boils and the sugar is dissolved. Reduce the heat and simmer for 4–5 minutes. Remove from the heat and cool. Stir in the flours and bicarbonate of soda. Fold in the nuts and mix well. Place in a large loaf or 20 cm-square tin, lined with greaseproof paper, and bake in a moderate oven for 50–60 minutes or until a skewer comes out clean.

Carob Fruit Loaf

No eggs, sugar or added fat. This is a good sweet treat for weight watchers!

1 cup mixed dried fruit
1 cup wheatgerm
1 1/4 cups soy, rice or skim milk
1/4 cup carob powder, sifted
1 cup wholemeal self-raising flour, sifted

Combine the dried fruit, wheatgerm and milk in a large bowl, then cover and stand for 2 hours in refrigerator. Fold in the carob and flour and mix well. Place in a greaseproof paper lined loaf tin and bake at 180°C for 45–60 minutes.

Carrot and Citrus Cake

3/4 cup white self-raising flour
3/4 cup wholemeal self-raising flour
1 cup raw sugar
1/2 teaspoon cinnamon powder
1 cup grated carrot
juice and grated zest of 1 small lemon
1/2 cup virgin cold-pressed olive oil
2 x 60 g eggs, beaten
1/2 cup chopped mixed peel
1 tablespoon brandy

Sift the flours into a large bowl, stir in sugar and cinnamon. Add the carrot, lemon zest and oil, then the eggs. Stir in the mixed peel and lemon juice, add the brandy and mix well. Place in an oiled and greasproof paper lined 20 cm cake tin. Sprinkle a little extra chopped mixed peel over the top and bake in the oven at 180°C for 1 1/4 hours or until a skewer comes out clean.

This cake contains plenty of antioxidants!

Pumpkin Fruit Cake

$^1/_2$ cup cold-pressed oil
1 cup brown sugar
$^3/_4$ cup white self-raising flour, sifted
$^3/_4$ cup wholemeal plain flour, sifted
2 x 60 g eggs, beaten
1 teaspoon vanilla essence
1 cup mashed cooked pumpkin
2 cups mixed dried fruit
LSA or chopped nuts, if desired

Place the oil and sugar in a saucepan and stir over a low heat until the sugar has melted. Mix in the remaining ingredients and pour into a lined 20 cm-cake tin. Sprinkle the top of the mixture with LSA (page 72) or chopped nuts and bake in a moderate oven for 1 hour or until a skewer comes out clean. This is a very moist cake.

Moist Coconut Pie (made in a jiffy!)

4 x 60 g eggs, lightly beaten
$^1/_2$ cup cold-pressed oil
$^3/_4$ cup plain wholemeal flour
$^1/_2$ cup raw sugar
1 cup dessicated coconut
400 g can coconut milk
1 tablespoon lemon juice

Blend all the ingredients together until smooth. Pour into a 23 cm-pie plate and bake in a moderate oven for 1 hour. Serve, just warm, with whipped tofu or Vitari ice cream and sprinkle with toasted coconut.

Rich Date and Brandy Pudding (delicious!)

$^3/_4$ cup chopped dates
1 teaspoon bicarbonate of soda
1 cup boiling water
$^1/_2$ cup virgin cold-pressed olive oil
1 cup brown sugar
2 x x 60 g eggs, beaten
1 cup wholemeal self-raising flour, sifted

Syrup

$^3/_4$ cup brown sugar
1 tablespoon honey
1 cup water
1 teaspoon vanilla essence
75 ml brandy

Soak the dates and bicarbonate of soda in the boiling water. Heat the oil, stir in the sugar over a low heat, cool, then beat in the eggs and fold in the flour. Add the date mixture and pour into an oiled 20 x 30 cm ovenproof dish. Bake in a moderate oven for 35–45 minutes.

To make the syrup: Boil together the sugar, honey and water until slightly thickened and syrupy. Remove from the heat, stir in the vanilla essence and brandy and leave to cool. Pour over the pudding as soon as it comes out of the oven. Serve immediately.

Frozen Apple and Pear Dessert

1 William or Packham pear, cored and unpeeled
1 granny smith apple, cored and unpeeled
½ cup soy, oat or skim milk
1 teaspoon honey
1 scoop Vitari ice cream
1 tablespoon gelatin, dissolved in a little hot water
400 g can coconut milk

Blend all the ingredients together in a food processor until smooth. Pour into a container and freeze. Serve in scoops with crushed almonds and poached pears.

Italian-style Nut Bread

3 egg whites
½ cup raw sugar
1 cup plain wholemeal flour
1 cup chopped hazelnuts (or any other unsalted nuts)
1 teaspoon vanilla extract

Whisk the egg whites until peaks form, then slowly beat in the sugar until the mixture thickens. Fold in the sifted flour, nuts and vanilla.

Spread the mixture into a very well oiled 25 x 8 cm bar tin. Bake in a moderate oven for about 30 minutes until firm. Remove from tin and cool. Wrap in foil and store for 1–2 days. Using a very sharp knife cut bread into wafer-thin slices. Place on a baking tray and bake in a slow oven for 30–40 minutes or until dry and crisp. Store in an airtight container!

Joyce's Date Slice

2 x 60 g eggs, separated
½ cup raw sugar
1 cup plain wholemeal flour, sifted
1 cup chopped pecan nuts
1 cup chopped, pitted dates

Whisk the egg whites until stiff, then fold in the sugar and whisk again. Whisk in the egg yolks. When the mixture thickens, fold in the sifted flour, nuts and dates. Spread the mixture onto a very well-oiled baking tray. Bake in a moderate oven until firm (about 30 minutes). Cut into slices while still warm. Allow to cool, then dust lightly with icing sugar.

Sesame & Coconut Confectionery

½ cup honey
½ cup ground sunflower seed kernels
1–2 cups very finely chopped dried apricots
1 cup sesame seeds
1½ cups desiccated coconut

Place the honey into a saucepan, bring to the boil and simmer for 2 minutes; cool. Stir in the sunflower seeds and apricots and boil gently for another minute. Add the sesame seeds and coconut, mix well. Press into a greased, paper-lined 28 cm square tin and refrigerate until set. Cut into squares.

Mostly Fruit Cake

1 cup glacé cherries or a mixture of chopped glacé fruit
2 cups chopped mixed nuts (pecans, almonds, hazelnuts)
$1\frac{1}{2}$ cups pitted dates
$\frac{3}{4}$ cup plain flour
$\frac{1}{2}$ teaspoon baking powder
$\frac{1}{2}$ cup raw sugar
3 x 60 g eggs
1 teaspoon vanilla

Preheat the oven to 150°C. Grease a 20 cm round cake tin and line with foil or greased paper. Place glacé fruit, nuts and whole dates in a bowl. Sift the flour and baking powder, into the bowl, add sugar and mix well. Beat the eggs until frothy, add the vanilla and stir into the mixture. When thoroughly combined, spread into prepared tin. Bake for $1\frac{3}{4}$ hours, remove from the tin, peel off the paper and cool. Wrap and store in the refrigerator. To serve, slice thinly.

Spice & Raisin Biscuits

2 cups raisins
1 large egg white
1 cup frozen unsweetened apple juice concentrate, thawed
3 tablespoons oil
$1\frac{1}{2}$ cups wholemeal plain flour
1 cup quick-cooking rolled oats
1 teaspoon baking powder
1 teaspoon cinnamon
1 teaspoon ground cloves

Place the raisins into a saucepan and just cover with water; boil gently for 10 minutes. Drain well and reserve the water. Mix the egg white, apple juice and oil into a bowl. Add the flour, oats, baking soda, cinnamon, and cloves; mix well. Add $\frac{1}{4}$ cup of reserved raisin water and stir through.

Place teaspoonful of the mixture onto a baking tray that has been sprayed with nonstick vegetable coating. Bake at 200°C for 10 minutes, or until lightly brown. Makes about 30.

Favourite Muffins

2 cups wholemeal plain flour, sifted
3 tablespoons LSA (page 72)
$\frac{1}{3}$ cup wheatgerm
$1\frac{1}{2}$ teaspoons baking soda
$\frac{1}{4}$ cup frozen unsweetened apple juice concentrate, thawed
$\frac{3}{4}$ cup frozen unsweetened pineapple juice concentrate, thawed
2 large egg whites
1 teaspoon vanilla
$\frac{1}{2}$ cup unsweetened crushed pineapple, drained
1 cup finely grated carrot

In a large bowl combine the sifted flour, LSA, wheatgerm, and baking soda. Combine juices, egg whites, vanilla, pineapple, and carrot and add to the dry ingredients. Stir until just moistened. Spoon the batter into a very well-oiled muffin tin or paper muffin cup inserts. Bake at 200°C for 15–20 minutes. Serve warm. Makes 12.

Patricia's Home-made Granola (for a sweet breakfast! Or even lunch!)

4 cups rolled oats
4 cups rolled wheat
1 cup fresh wheatgerm
1–2 cups slivered almonds, optional
¾ cup frozen unsweetened apple juice concentrate, thawed
2 teaspoons vanilla
4 tablespoons LSA (page 72)
¾ cup dried apples, cut into bite-sized pieces
¾ cup chopped dates
¾ cup raisins
1 cup raw sunflower seeds

Mix together the oats, rolled wheat and wheatgerm, adding almonds, if desired. Combine the apple juice and vanilla and add to the oat mixture, blending well. Pour into a lightly oiled 22 x 32 cm pan and bake at 120°–150°C for 1 hour. Adjust the temperature for your oven and be careful if you use a fan forced oven. After taking the granola out of the oven, add the LSA, dried apples, dates, raisins and sunflower seeds. Makes about 12 cups. Serve with oat, rice or soy milk.

ARTIFICIAL SWEETENERS

During my widespread travels I am continually shocked by the large number of people still consuming artificial sweeteners, especially the highly toxic sweetener, aspartame. These artificial sweeteners must be broken down by the detoxification systems in the liver and increase the workload of the liver much more than natural sugars.

If you increase the workload of the liver's detoxification systems, you will use up valuable energy in the liver cells, that is required for fat metabolism. Thus your ability to burn fat will be compromised and you will gain weight more easily. This explains why artificial sweeteners do not help those with weight excess, indeed they are fattening.

Aspartame is a molecule composed of three components—aspartic acid, phenylalanine and methanol. Once broken down by the liver, the methanol (wood alcohol) converts into formaldehyde and formic acid (ant-sting poison). Formaldehyde, a deadly neurotoxin, is a common embalming fluid and a class A carcinogen.

Aspartame is a commonly used artificial sweetener.

Some people have suffered aspartame related disorders with doses as small as that carried in a single stick of chewing gum. Pilots who drink diet sodas may be more susceptible to flicker vertigo, flicker-induced epileptic activity, sudden memory loss, dizziness during instrument flight and gradual loss of vision. Some pilots have experienced *grand mal* seizures in the cockpits of commercial airline flights and have lost medical certification to fly.

The FDA has received more than 10,000 consumer complaints about artificial sweeteners. That's 80 per cent of all complaints about food additives, yet they remain comatose and have done nothing to alert the American public who assume that since it's so highly advertised, it must be safe.

If you are using aspartame and have headaches, depression, slurred speech, loss of memory, fibromyalgia-type symptoms, loss of sensation in lower legs or shooting pains, loss of equilibrium, vertigo, anxiety attacks, chronic fatigue, vision loss, seizures or heart palpitations, you may have ASPARTAME DISEASE! Many physicians are diagnosing multiple sclerosis (MS) when in reality it is methanol toxicity caused by aspartame which mimics MS.

Researchers at Massachusetts Institute of Technology surveyed 80 people who suffered brain seizures after eating or drinking products with Aspartame. The Community Nutrition Institute states—'These 80 cases meet the FDA's own definition of an imminent hazard to public health, which requires the FDA to expeditiously remove a product from the market'.

Pregnant women or those trying to conceive should avoid artificial sweeteners. Foetal tissue cannot tolerate methanol, and Dr James Bowen calls NutraSweet instant birth control. The foetal placenta can concentrate phenylalanine which may increase the risk of mental retardation. Aspartame tests on animals produced brain and mammary tumors.

During Operation Desert Storm, truckloads of diet drinks cooked in the Arabian sun. Aspartame liberates methanol in the can! Thousands of service men and women returned home with chronic fatigue syndrome and weird toxic symptoms!

Aspartame and other artificial sweeteners make you crave carbohydrates so you gain weight. They do not help diabetics although millions of diabetics are using aspartame products.

Dr H. J. Roberts (world expert on Aspartame and diabetic specialist) says 'I now advise ALL patients with diabetes and hypoglycemia to avoid Aspartame products.'

Neurosurgeon, Russell Blaylock, MD, in his book entitled *EXCITOTOXINS—THE TASTE THAT KILLS*, says Aspartame may trigger clinical diabetes! He states that, 'What really concerns me about aspartame is its association with brain tumors as well as pancreatic, uterine and ovarian tumors and that so many develop an Alzheimer's-like syndrome with prolonged exposure'.

Artificial sweeteners are dangerous toxins in our society because of their ubiquitous presence in thousands of foods, even children's vitamins and medicine and are found on every restaurant table and in every hotel/motel room.

References:

H. J. ROBERTS, MD, FACP, FCCP. Books and publications:

Aspartame: Is it Safe? The Charles Press, PO Box 15715S, Philadelphia PA 19103.

Much of this information was prepared from facts and statistics collected by the organisation MISSION POSSIBLE, PO BOX 28098, Atlanta, GA 30358 USA. For further information on aspartame e-mail betty@pd.org and put as the subject line 'sendme help'.

ALTERNATIVE SAFE AND NATURAL SWEETENERS

The natural sugars on the list below provide an easily digested and quick form of energy to the cells.

date sugar
maple sugar or syrup
rice syrup
molasses
honey
fruit jams
raw sugar
carob
dried fruits
fresh fruit, fruit juices and fruit juice concentrates
Stevia, a sweet tasting herb. (However it may be difficult to obtain Stevia in Australia from anywhere other than multi-level marketing companies, which makes it rather expensive.)

Natural sources of sugar such as fruit, honey, maple syrup, barley malt, carob, date sugar and unrefined granulated sugar cane juice contain adequate supplies of minerals and vitamins, which are essential for the metabolism of sugar. These are preferable to refined forms of sugar.

Honey as well as being a good sweetener has other health benefits. Honey is good for the digestion, is an antibiotic and a natural tranquilliser and according to several of my patients it has helped to lower their blood pressure.

Carob, a natural sweetener with a chocolatey-type flavour, contains B vitamins and minerals. Carob is found in tablet, syrup, powder, bars and wafer forms. Carob may be used as a substitute for chocolate or cocoa in those with allergies or sensitivities to caffeine.

All sugars can be harmful if they are eaten to excess, when they can lead to obesity which may increase the risk of diabetes. However, if natural sugars are eaten in small amounts they are able to boost both energy and the enjoyment of life. I do not think that totally sugar-free diets are healthy and, furthermore, they do not work in the long term because people feel deprived and miserable and cannot stick to them.

CHAPTER SIX

OVERCOMING CHRONIC FATIGUE SYNDROME

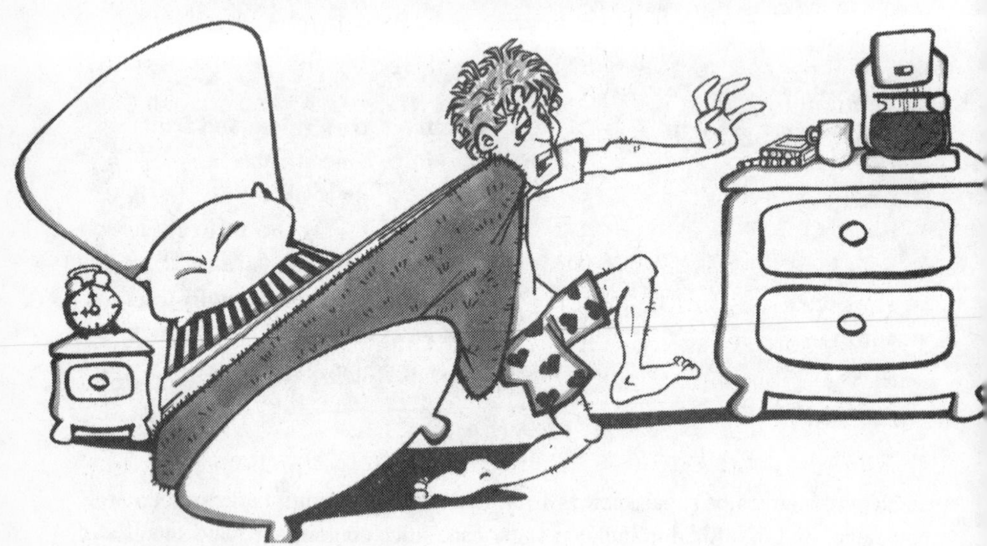

If you do not feel well in the mornings and drag yourself out of bed, looking for coffee, sugar, cigarettes and other stimulants, then your adrenal glands may be underactive.

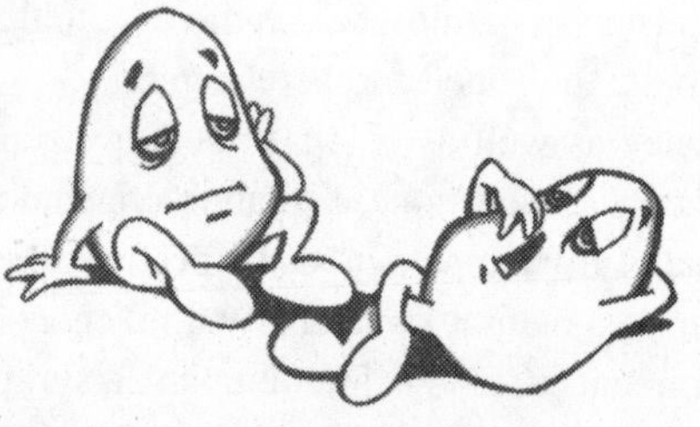

For many years it has been difficult for patients with 'chronic fatigue syndrome' to gain recognition for their illness, let alone effective treatment. Some have endured expensive and often unpleasant investigations and tests, only to be told that they have a psychosomatic disorder, such as depression, neurosis, stress or hypochondriasis. Thankfully, the definition for chronic fatigue syndrome (CFS) was recently specified by the Centre for Disease Control in the USA, which was a relief for many patients who thought that they were slowly going crazy.

The accepted definition of CFS is fatigue which persists for more than six months. Commonly associated symptoms are muscular pains, lymph gland swelling and recurrent viral infections.

The fatigue in these patients is actually a message to the body that the patient must rest in order to stop more damage occurring. In these patients the immune system is overloaded and is in a state of continual excitation with the production of excessive inflammatory chemicals.

The production of toxic, free radicals is excessive and damages the energy factories (mitochondria) within our cells. These free radicals, inflammatory chemicals and viral particles, attack musculo-skeletal tissues and the lymph nodes, causing aches and pains and glandular swellings.

Allergies and chemical sensitivities often supervene in these patients because their immune system is so overloaded and 'hyped up'. As a result, the body shuts down and goes into a state of metabolic hybernation for the purpose of self-preservation.

CFS can affect people of all ages and often follows a long period during which the patient has been repeatedly subjected to immune stressors—i.e. emotional stress, exposure to toxic chemicals or addictive drugs, multiple and frequent vaccinations, incorrect diet and food allergies, infections, overuse of antibiotic drugs, overuse of anti-inflammatory drugs, use of steroid drugs.

At the convention of the American College of Advancement in Medicine (ACAM) in 1992, the general consensus of the speakers was that CFS is probably not caused by one factor alone but is due to a combination of infectious viruses. Blood tests in these patients often show non-specific immune deficiencies. The most common viruses to trigger CFS are the family of herpes viruses, such as Epstein-Barr virus (glandular fever virus) and herpes VI virus. The virus that causes chicken pox and shingles and the cytomegalovirus can also be incriminated. These viruses are very common and 90 per cent of the population has contacted Epstein-Barr virus by the time of young adulthood. If your immune system is healthy and strong these viruses will be easily overthrown and most people carry these viruses in a dormant or quiescent state during their lives. If this was not so, the entire population would have CFS.

In CFS victims who carry these viruses, the problem is not the virus *per se*, it is the fact that the weakened immune system has become overloaded and cannot keep the virus in an inactive state. Many people with CFS become confused and blame their illness on a specific virus; however, the problem is the immune system and it is the immune system that we must concentrate on and not the virus. There is no safe way to kill all the viral particles and viral DNA in your body and we need to strengthen the immune system which will then keep the viruses in an inactive and harmless form.

The path to recovery from CFS is often slow; however, if patients follow a three-step plan a gradual recovery usually occurs and a complete cure is often the outcome.

THREE-STEP PLAN TO RECOVERY FROM CFS

STEP 1

TAKE THE LOAD OFF THE IMMUNE SYSTEM

The most effective way to do this is through the liver because the liver is intimately related to the immune system. The liver is the cleansing filter of the bloodstream and if it performs this function efficiently, your bloodstream will be much healthier; the blood cells will be in better condition and there will be less toxic chemicals, waste products, inflammatory chemicals, undesirable fats and micro-organisms present in the plasma (fluid) part of the bloodstream. Therefore, your immune system will not have to cope with these unwanted blood contaminants and its workload will be less.

I have seen time and time again that if one improves liver function the workload of the immune system is reduced and it is then possible for the immune system to rest and rejuvenate itself. The previously overactive immune system then quietens down as it is no longer in a state of continual war and it gradually stops producing excessive amounts of inflammatory chemicals which exacerbate CFS.

To improve liver function it is necessary to **follow a liver-cleansing diet** and I have written a whole book on this subject. If you have CFS I urge you to try this diet for at least three months (see *The Liver-Cleansing Diet* book by Dr Sandra Cabot, published by the WHAS 1996).

The principles of the liver-cleansing diet are:

1. Eat more raw food (raw fruit and/or vegetables with every meal). Thirty to 40 per cent of the diet should consist of raw fruit and vegetables.
2. Minimise consumption of high-fat dairy products (e.g. butter, hard cheese or cheese spreads, cream cheese, camembert cheese, cream, chocolate, ice cream).
3. Avoid damaged fats (e.g. deep-fried foods, margarines, processed fats, snack foods, takeaway fast foods, hydrogenated vegetable oils, oils that are not fresh).
4. Avoid artificial chemicals (e.g. artificial sweeteners, such as aspartame, colourings, flavourings, preservatives).
5. Eat an abundance of the good fats or essential fatty acids (e.g. cold-pressed seed and vegetable oils, avocados, fish, flaxseed, raw seeds and fresh raw nuts, legumes).
6. Consume a diverse source of proteins (e.g. from grains, nuts, seeds, legumes, free-range chicken, seafood, fish, free-range eggs and lean fresh red meat occasionally, if desired).
7. Eat lots of fruit and vegetables. Some of the vegetables may be cooked.
8. Use natural sugars (e.g. honey, molasses, dried fruit, fresh fruit, Vitari ice cream, fruit shakes made with soy, oat or rice milk).
9. Take plenty of fluids (e.g. water, raw juices, herbal teas and weak regular tea if desired). Aim for 2 litres daily. This is vitally important.

The fourteen-day energy diet given on pages 76 to 93, has many similarities to the Liver-Cleansing Diet but for more in-depth understanding and variety I suggest you read my *Liver-Cleansing Diet* book. The key to a healthy liver is by correct diet and, thankfully, the liver has remarkable powers of repair and regeneration.

Since writing my *Liver-Cleansing Diet* book I have received thousands of letters from participants and readers. Some have followed this diet just because they wanted to be healthier, while many have followed it because of poor health. I have many testimonies from those who had liver diseases, auto-immune diseases, chronic fatigue, obesity and/or fatty liver and these give factual evidence that these problems can be greatly helped and often cured by following a diet specifically to improve the liver.

If your liver function is sluggish and your liver is overburdened with toxins, you will feel tired, bloated and moody and may suffer with headaches and allergies. You may become 'allergic to the twentieth century' and intolerant of many chemicals and foods because your liver has stopped producing the enzymes that detoxify chemicals and drugs. If you are exposed to these things you may have a violent reaction because your overloaded inefficient liver can no longer protect you. Living in this day and age it is not possible to have a 'squeaky clean' environment and, anyway, we need a small amount of chemicals to induce the liver to keep making its detoxifying enzymes. This is the reason why salicylate intolerant people often do better on a low-salicylate diet than on a no-salicylate diet.

Liver overload, dysfunction and fatty liver are the result of the modern Western diet which burdens the liver with excess unhealthy fats, animal protein, refined carbohydrates and toxic chemicals. If we have an unbalanced excessive diet, the more toxic nitrogenous by-products the liver has to break down, the more tired we become.

Liver Tonics

For those with an overburdened liver I recommend using a liver tonic that contains a mixture of liver herbs and the amino acid taurine.

Taurine plays several important roles in the body and is an essential component of cell membranes where it stabilises transport across the cell membrane and gives anti-oxidant protection. Taurine plays a major role in the liver via the formation of bile acids and detoxification. Abnormally low levels of taurine are common in many patients with chemical sensitivities and allergies. Taurine is the major amino acid required by the liver for the removal of toxic chemicals and metabolites from the body. It is required for the conjugation of drugs and metabolites in the liver via the acylation route. Once conjugated, chemical toxins are removed from the body as a component of the bile and also through water-soluble acetates in the urine. Taurine is a key component of bile acids produced in the liver. Taurine is the body's main anti-oxidant defence against production of excess hypochlorite ion which can lead to severe chemical sensitivities if it is not controlled. Impaired body synthesis of taurine will reduce the ability of the liver to detoxify environmental chemicals such as chlorine, chlorite (bleach), aldehydes (produced from alcohol excess), alcohol, petroleum solvents and ammonia. Taurine is one of the major nutrients involved in the liver's detoxification of harmful substances and drugs and can help chemically sensitive patients. Taurine is found in animal protein, organ meats and seafood and is often deficient in vegetarians or those with inflammatory bowel diseases. All good liver tonic powders and capsules should contain taurine. Factors that increase the body's taurine needs are strict vegetarianism, epilepsy, fad diets, alcohol, oral contraceptives, cortisone therapy, high stress levels and a high intake of MSG.

My favourite herbs for the liver are dandelion, St Mary's thistle and globe artichoke and I have had very good results using these herbs in those with fatty liver, obesity and liver dysfunction. All good liver tonic powders and capsules should contain these three herbs along with taurine.

Dandelion has been used for centuries to treat liver and biliary complaints and today is still used widely as a liver tonic in North

America, Australia, Europe and the Orient. The therapeutic properties of dandelion are due in part to its bitter substances taraxacin and inulin (a bitter glycoside). Other active substances in dandelion are sesquiterpenes, flavonoids, levulin, fatty acids, minerals and vitamins. Bitters, such as those in dandelion, stimulate the digestive glands and the liver and activate the flow of bile. *The Australian Journal of Medical Herbalism* Vol 3 (4), 1991, refers to two studies, which demonstrate the liver healing properties of dandelion. They found that dandelion successfully treats hepatitis, liver swelling, jaundice and indigestion in those with inadequate bile secretion. As well as in the form of a liver tonic, dandelion can be consumed as the fresh dandelion greens in salads.

St Mary's thistle (also known as milk thistle or *Silybum marianum*) has been known as a traditional liver tonic for centuries and more than 100 scientific research papers have been produced on its liver healing properties. (Reference 2.)

St Mary's thistle has multiple actions; these are liver protective, liver regenerative and anti-oxidant. It can be used with benefit in the following liver problems: chronic hepatitis, cirrhosis, liver damage, bile stagnation and alcohol and chemical induced fatty liver. St Mary's thistle has been found to reduce toxic fatty degeneration of the liver. Clinical and laboratory studies and tissue examinations, both in humans and animals have found St Mary's thistle to be of benefit in treating all of the above. The powerful liver detoxification enzymes that break down drugs and toxic chemicals are called the cytochrome P450 enzymes. These enzymes are improved by one of the components of St Mary's thistle called silibinin. All good liver tonics should contain St Mary's thistle.

Globe artichoke *(Cynara scolymus)* has liver protective and restorative actions. In overweight people it can be used to lower elevated cholesterol and triglycerides. It is also a good 'blood cleanser' for those with skin diseases, bad breath and body odour. All good liver tonic powders and capsules should contain globe artichoke. For more information on liver tonics call a naturopath on (09) 478 5921 in New Zealand

THE LIVER AND DETOXIFICATION

The liver is the gateway to the body and in this day and age has an enormous workload that may overload its detoxification systems. The liver must try to cope with every toxic chemical in our food chain and environment, as well as excessive amounts of damaged fats that are present in fast foods.

Let us examine the ways by which the liver keeps our internal body clean and healthy.

THE LIVER FILTER

If we examine the liver filter under a microscope we see rows of liver cells separated by spaces called sinusoids. Sinusoids are structured

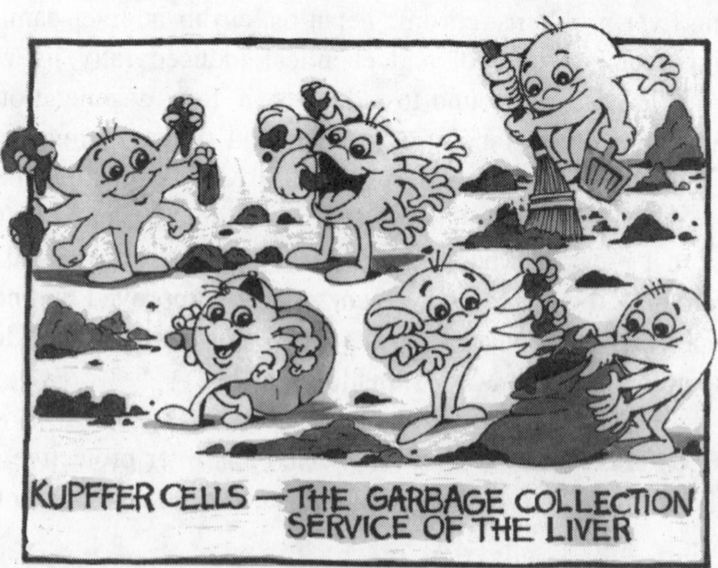

like a filter or sieve through which the bloodstream flows. During this process the sinusoidal filter removes toxic matter (such as particles, micro-organisms, dead cells and waste products) from the bloodstream. Once captured inside the sinusoidal filter, these noxious things are ingested by specialised cells called Kupffer cells. A Kupffer cell looks like a tiny octopus and is very efficient in wrapping and ingesting foreign bodies. Once the Kupffer cell has its dangerous victim inside of it, it then breaks it down into harmless substances. The sinusoids and Kupffer cells are like a complete 'garbage disposal unit' within the liver. Thus, you can see that the liver is of vital importance as the filter and cleanser of the bloodstream.

THE LIVER DETOXIFICATION PATHWAY

Inside the liver cells (hepatocytes) there are sophisticated chemical pathways, that have evolved over millions of years, to break down toxic substances. Every drug, artificial chemical, pesticide and hormone is broken down or metabolised by these pathways inside the liver cells. Basically there are two major detoxification pathways inside the liver cells which are called the Phase One and Phase Two Detoxification Pathways.

Phase One Detoxification Pathway

This is called the Cytochrome P450 enzyme system whereby a toxic chemical is changed into a less harmful substance. This is achieved by various chemical reactions such as oxidation, reduction, hydrolysis or hydroxylation. During this process, oxygen free radicals are generated which can damage the liver cells. Vitamin C is the most effective way to prevent these free radicals from causing cellular damage. If vitamin C is lacking, toxic chemicals will become far more dangerous.

Phase Two Detoxification Pathway

This is called the conjugation pathway, whereby the liver cells add either a glycine or sulphate molecule to a toxic chemical or drug. This makes the toxin or drug water soluble, so it is then able to be eliminated from the body via fluids, such as urine or bile. Through conjugation the liver is able to turn drugs, hormones and various toxins into excretable substances. For efficient phase two detoxification the liver cells require sulphur-containing amino acids such as taurine, methionine and cysteine. The nutrients glycine, glutamine, choline and inositol are also required for efficient phase two detoxification. Cruciferous vegetables (cabbage, broccoli, cauliflower, brussels sprouts) are a good source of natural sulphur compounds to help the phase two detoxification pathway. Thus, these vegetables can be considered cleansing foods.

If the phase one and phase two detoxification pathways become overloaded there will be a build up of various toxins in the body. Many of these toxins are fat soluble and incorporate themselves into the fatty parts of the body where they may stay for years, if not a lifetime. Because the brain and endocrine glands are fatty organs, they are common sites for fat-soluble toxins to accumulate. This may result in symptoms of brain dysfunction and hormonal imbalances. Many of these chemicals (such as pesticides, petrochemicals, aspartame etc.) are carcinogenic and have been implicated in the rising incidence of many cancers. If the filtering and/or detoxification systems within the liver are overloaded or inefficient, this will cause toxins, dead cells and micro-organisms to build up in the bloodstream. This will then increase the workload of the immune system which may become overloaded and hyper-stimulated. This may lead to symptoms of immune dysfunction such as allergies, inflammatory states, swollen glands, recurrent infections, auto-immune diseases or chronic fatigue syndrome.

These disorders are very common in the chemically overloaded environment we live in today and are usually treated by drugs to suppress these symptoms. Rarely does anyone think about the liver, which is unfortunate because the simplest and most effective way to take the load off the immune system, is to help the liver to work more efficiently. To improve liver function I suggest you follow my liver-cleansing diet (see page 110) and take a liver tonic (see page 111). Also, ensure that you are obtaining sufficient vitamin C by eating foods that are abundant in this vitamin (see page 133).

Many people believe that it is important to cleanse and detoxify the bowels with herbal laxatives and enemas or colonic irrigations. This may be helpful; however, it is important to understand that the bowels are not able to cleanse the bloodstream or remove debris from the cells. It is far more important to keep your liver healthy because it is the first line of defence against toxins and micro-organisms in our food and water supplies. These and other environmental toxins pose a big threat to our immune system.

If these toxins are not dealt with effectively by the liver, they accumulate in our bodies and this is a big reason for the deteriorating health of people as they age. The oestrogenic effect of pesticides is a significant factor in the worldwide epidemic of breast cancer. It is vital to support liver function with nutritional medicine if we are to protect ourselves from these toxic pollutants. I also encourage the use of household water filters to reduce toxins and micro-organisms in the water supply. The best types of water filters are those with submicron-solid carbon-block filters as they are able to remove parasites. Parasitic infections, such as giardia, cryptosporidium and amoeba and other bowel parasites can cause ill health and liver damage. Another important strategy is to encourage the growth of organic agriculture and chemical-free food. Many health food stores now stock drug- and hormone-free animal proteins.

STEP 2

STRENGTHEN THE IMMUNE SYSTEM WITH NUTRIENTS

THE FORGOTTEN MINERALS

Many patients with chronic fatigue syndrome (CFS) are mineral deficient. This is because the soils and therefore food chain is often mineral depleted, processed foods and fast foods are mineral deficient, diuretics, coffee and alcohol excess cause mineral losses, certain drugs reduce mineral absorption and utilisation and digestive problems and inflammatory bowel diseases reduce mineral absorption.

It is difficult to test for deficiencies of many trace minerals as they are mostly found **inside** the cells, muscles, soft tissues and bones and only a very small percentage is floating around in the bloodstream. For example, if a blood test is done to measure the serum and red blood cell magnesium level, only less than 1 per cent of the total body magnesium is being checked, as the rest is inacessible.

Clues that you may be mineral deficient are: fatigue, low blood sugar and sugar cravings, muscle twitches and spasms, diseases of cardiac muscle or skeletal muscle, dizziness, light headedness, thyroid underactivity and hair loss.

MAGNESIUM

Let us start with the mineral **magnesium** which I have found to be of great help to those with CFS. Magnesium is known to be essentially involved in the production of energy and activates five groups of major enzymes. It performs a critical role in the activation of four of the nine enzymes in the tri-carboxylic acid cycle (TCA cycle). The TCA cycle is at the **very centre of all cellular metabolism** involving protein, fat and carbohydrate metabolism.

Magnesium has a crucial role in the external and internal cell membranes where it enables transfer of **electro-chemical energy.**

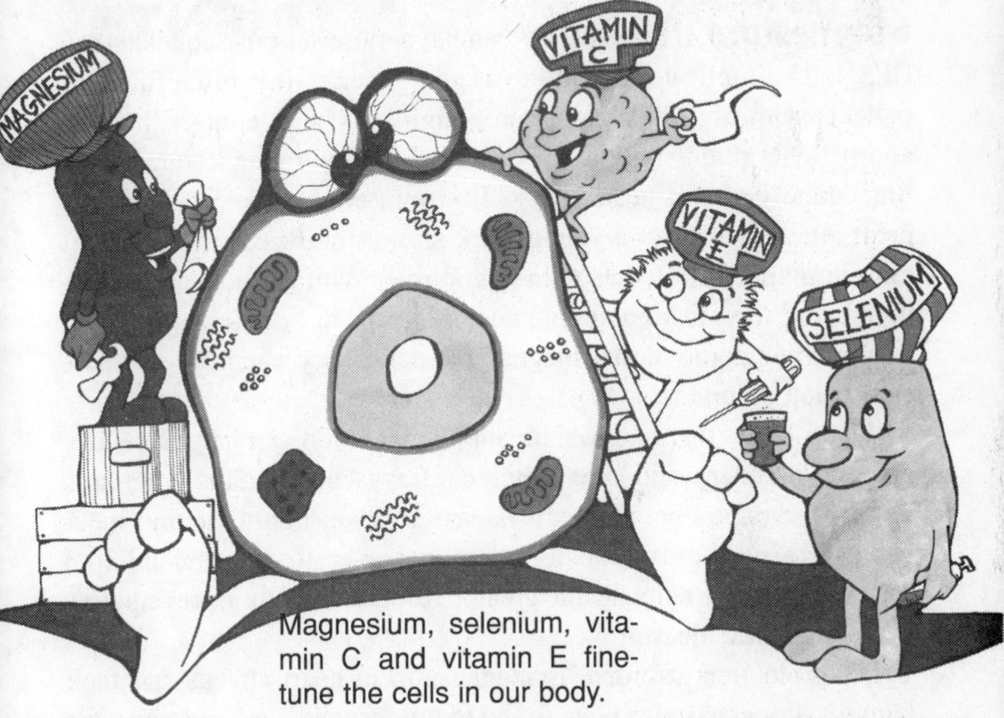

Magnesium, selenium, vitamin C and vitamin E fine-tune the cells in our body.

Magnesium has a regulating effect upon the entire **nervous system** and controls neuronal activity and excitability, overall having a **relaxing effect.**

Magnesium is essential for **cell growth and repair** being needed for protein manufacture, the manufacture of genetic material (DNA) and ATP (energy) metabolism. It is a **master mineral** in that it co-ordinates the proper function of nerves, muscle, blood vessels, bone, calcium metabolism and the chemical stability of the central nervous system.

Magnesium plays a crucial role at the heart of cellular metabolism. It is not surprising that a deficiency of magnesium, even of a slight degree, could seriously reduce the body's production of energy and prevent recovery from CFS.

Magnesium deficiency can have more serious sequelae than CFS and is implicated in cardiovascular disease. It is often found in patients with high blood pressure, angina or heart attacks (infarct) and patients often show a marked drop in blood magnesium levels immediately after a heart attack. Post-mortem studies in victims of heart attacks (often at a young age), show significantly lower heart muscle magnesium levels than in controls. With cardiovascular disease being the most common cause of death in both sexes by far, I think it is imperative that magnesium deficiency is considered as a significant culprit.

We do know that magnesium supplementation can help to reduce the risk of sudden and unexpected cardiovascular dealths, often at a relatively young age, and as it is easy to give, non-toxic and inexpensive this should make us all more eager to recommend it. I believe it should demand far greater respect as both a preventative and therapeutic measure.

The protection afforded by magnesium in heart attacks and their complications, has also been found to hold true in stroke victims and migraine sufferers where spasm of the cerebral arteries is occurring. **Migraine sufferers are often lacking magnesium** as determined by nuclear magnetic resonance spectroscopy.

Testing for magnesium deficiency is difficult because a blood test to measure serum magnesium only assesses 1 per cent of the total body content. Normal serum levels are 0.7–1.0 mmol/litre = 1.4–1.9 meq/l.

One can measure the magnesium levels inside the red blood cells to get a slightly better idea of possible deficiency. Normal red blood cell levels of magnesium are 5.2–7.5 mmol/litre. These tests are guidelines only and one should also be guided by symptoms of magnesium deficiency because red blood cell and serum levels of magnesium only test 1 per cent of the total body magnesium. It is also possible to measure magnesium in a twenty-four-hour collection of urine if the laboratory is notified ahead of time.

Magnesium deficiency is quite common, affecting over 40 per cent of people with high blood pressure, 65 per cent of patients with congestive heart failure and 36–75 per cent of the general population.

The Recommended Daily Allowance (RDA) of magnesium described in the USA in 1980 is as follows:

Category	Milligrams per day
Female over 11 years	300
Pregnant or lactating female	450
Male	350–400
Children	50–250

The RDA amounts are often underestimates as they are given as the amounts to prevent disease and are not given for optimum health. The RDAs do not take individual body weights, stress levels, family history or metabolism into account either. Many so-called 'healthy' people do not even obtain this low RDA. It is not uncommon to find people who consume 25–50 per cent less magnesium than the controversial RDA. There has been a 50 per cent reduction in the dietary intake of magnesium in the USA over the last eighty years which probably reflects the higher consumption of processed foods over this time. The common lack of magnesium in the Western diet is compounded by the fact that a diet high in dairy products and sugar raises the daily requirements for magnesium to between 500 and 800 milligrams.

We know that blood pressure tends to be higher in groups with a low magnesium intake. Vegetarians consume more magnesium from nuts, beans, legumes, unprocessed cereals and green leafy vegetables which partially explains why they have a lower incidence of high blood pressure and heart disease.

The ratio of calcium to magnesium in the diet, water supply or through supplementation is also important, especially because of the large number of women taking calcium supplements. The incidence of cardiovascular disease is higher if the ratio of calcium to magnesium exceeds 2:1. Finland has one of the highest incidences of cardiovascular disease and the ratio of calcium to magnesium in the water supply is 4:1. The ratio in the USA is 3:1. We need to be more conservative in the big rush to get women to have very high calcium intakes of around 1200 to 1500 mg daily, because with an average daily magnesium intake of only 250–300 mg, we are producing calcium to magnesium ratios of between 4:1 and 5:1.

Foods rich in magnesium are:

nuts (almonds, brazils, cashews, peanuts, pecans, walnuts, pistachio) soy beans, unprocessed grains (barley, millet, oats, rye, wild rice, corn) vegetables (especially parsnips, beet, leafy greens, peas, carrots,) kelp, brewers yeast, molasses, cocoa, chocolate (can you believe your luck!).

Possible signs of magnesium deficiency are:

high blood pressure, palpitations, vascular spasm, cold hands and feet, chest pains, shortness of breath, poor exercise tolerance, anxiety, agitation, irritability, insomnia, confusion, poor balance, muscular spasm and twitches, muscular weakness, muscular aches and pains, toxaemia of pregnancy, hyperactivity, kidney stones, increased tendency to epileptic convulsions.

Factors which increase the daily requirement for magnesium are:

stress, high muscular activity, high protein diets, processed foods, high calcium intake, many drugs such as diuretics, chemotherapy, antibiotics, excess alcohol and coffee.

After assessing hundreds of patients with chronic fatigue syndrome I am convinced that supplementation with magnesium can help greatly to speed up the rehabilitation process. Indeed, many of these patients would never recover without taking a good quality magnesium supplement every day.

The absorption of magnesium from the gut is very variable, depending upon many factors. It is known that between 40 and 70 per cent of ingested magnesium passes out through the faeces and so the majority may be lost. For this reason I recommend magnesium supplements that contain a mixture of various types of magnesium (e.g. magnesium phosphate, amino acid chelate, aspartate and orotate) to facilitate absorption from the gut into the bloodstream.

OTHER VITAL NUTRIENTS FOR CHRONIC FATIGUE

Those with chronic fatigue syndrome will benefit greatly from supplemental amounts of the most **essential minerals** plus anti-oxidants for the **immune system.** These are able to enhance **energy production** from the **mitochondria.** The mitochondria are the microscopic membranous energy factories found inside every cell in the body. If the mitochondria are not working efficiently the body's production of energy will be inadequate.

We find that today many people complain of mysterious **chronic fatigue** syndrome and are unable to find a solution. I have found that in the majority of chronic fatigue syndrome victims there are deficiencies of essential trace minerals and anti-oxidants.

Remember also that your bones require trace minerals along with calcium and indeed these trace minerals are just as important as calcium in the prevention of osteoporosis.

If you are deficient in trace minerals you are more likely to feel tired, moody, crave sugar and suffer with aches and pains.

Trace minerals are vitally important for the immune system and are needed for the body to effectively control viral infections.

Some minerals such as **selenium** and zinc are anti-inflammatory and are of great assistance in reducing skin diseases.

I have found that a special **designer yeast powder** that contains essential trace minerals such as **selenium, boron, chromium,** and **molybdenum** is of great benefit in those with chronic fatigue. It also provides the minerals zinc, manganese, calcium and magnesium. This powder also contains **anti-oxidants** from carrot, beetroot and barley grass powder, mixed tocopherols to provide the full range of **vitamin E** isomers and **vitamin C** in the form of ascorbic acid to provide extra anti-oxidant capability. **Lecithin** is added to boost phospholipids which are good for brain function and memory. **Alfalfa** provides a cleansing effect and contains beneficial phyto-sterols. The herb **kelp** is added to provide a broad spectrum of micro-minerals which are beneficial for the thyroid gland and the immune system. **Maleic acid** is added to enhance the energy-boosting properties.
For more information on designer yeast powders, call (02) 4653 1445 in Australia or (09) 478 5921 in New Zealand.

This type of yeast is very beneficial for nutritional health and just as there are both good and bad bacteria in the body, there are good and bad yeasts.

The good yeasts in powder form will enhance nutrition and immunity, whereas the bad yeasts (pathogenic yeasts), such as candida will overload the immune system.

Maleic acid is a natural substance derived from food sources or supplements and is synthesised in the body through the citric acid cycle. **It is vital for the production of energy in the mitochondria during both aerobic and anaerobic states.** Supplemental maleic acid can enhance the function of the mitochondria which may help those with **chronic fatigue** syndrome. The importance of maleic acid in the body's energy production is well established. Chronic fatigue **syndrome** is commonly associated with **fibromyalgia** which manifests as generalised musculo-skeletal pain, headache, stiffness, aching and tender localised spots in the muscles.

Maleic acid supplementation may be of use in improving energy production in fibromyalgia and its associated conditions. Maleic acid is of use as a supplement to boost levels of maleic acid within the cells to maintain an optimal level of energy production. (Reference 20.) A good quality designer yeast powder should contain maleic acid plus all the eight essential amino acids required for healthy metabolism.

Boron is a vitally important trace mineral required for the metabolism of calcium, phosphorous and magnesium. Boron deficiency will worsen vitamin D deficiency. For these reasons boron helps to prevent postmenopausal **osteoporosis** and builds muscle. A study conducted by the US Department of Agriculture indicated that within eight days of supplementing the daily diet with boron, a test group of postmenopausal women lost 40 per cent less calcium and one third less magnesium in their urine than before beginning boron supplementation. (Reference 21.) Boron improves brain function and increases alertness. Boron is present in some designer yeast powders and is well absorbed from such a source. It is also found in carrots, apples, leafy vegetables, grains, pears, nuts and grapes.

The essential mineral **molybdenum** is required in small amounts for protein, carbohydrate and fat metabolism. It promotes normal cellular function and is a component of cellular enzymes. A low intake of molybdenum is associated with mouth and gum disorders and cancer and may reduce sexual performance. Molybdenum supplementation can help those with **chronic fatigue** due to the overuse of antibiotics and candida infestation. It has also been found to reduce muscular pain, headaches, poor concentration and depression. (References 22 and 23.) Molybdenum is found in some designer yeast powders and green leafy vegetables, beans, legumes and cereal grains.

The mineral **chromium** is sometimes called the glucose tolerance factor because it is involved in the control of glucose (sugar) metabolism. This essential mineral maintains **stable blood sugar levels** by improving the utilisation of insulin and can help those with hypoglycaemia and diabetes. Studies have shown that low blood chromium levels can be an indication of coronary artery disease. Chromium is also needed for the metabolism of cholesterol, fats and protein. A deficiency of chromium can be associated with glucose intolerance, disturbed protein metabolism and increased risk of arterial disease. Chromium is helpful for those with **chronic fatigue** due to unstable blood sugar levels and sugar addiction. Processed and refined foods are extremely low or devoid of chromium. (References 24, 25, 26.) Chromium is found in some designer yeast powders, brewers yeast, meat, whole grains, brown rice, molasses, liver, chicken, corn, beans, eggs, potatoes and mushrooms. Herbs that contain chromium are yarrow, wild yam, red clover, oat straw, nettle, horsetail, liquorice, catnip and sarsparilla.

SELENIUM

The mineral Selenium is vital for the healthy function of the immune system. Some have called selenium the 'viral birth control pill' because of its ability to help those with recurrent viral illness. Beck and colleagues have shown that relatively harmless viruses can become virulent by passing through a selenium deficient host. (Reference 27.) **Selenium deficiency** has been shown in several studies to have adverse effects on susceptibility to many other disorders including cardiovascular disease and **cancer.** (Reference 28.) Those with a **strong family history of cancer,** especially **breast cancer,** would be wise to ensure adequate **selenium** intake. A study reported in *JAMA* (Reference 29) supports the hypothesis that supplemental selenium may reduce the incidence of, and mortality from, cancers of several sites.

Selenium also exerts a significant **anti-inflammatory effect** which is helpful for skin problems, musculo-skeletal inflammation and auto-immune dysfunction. Indeed, just about any chronic inflammatory process involving the body's most important organs, such as the heart, liver, kidneys, lungs and endocrine glands should be treated with supplemental selenium. **Selenium** is a **vital anti-oxidant** and reduces free radical damage of the **fatty membranes** and **genetic material** (DNA) inside the cells. This is partly due to its role in the intracellular anti-oxidant glutathione peroxidase enzymes.

Selenium, especially when combined with vitamin E, protects the immune system by preventing the formation of free radicals which damage body tissues and accelerate ageing.

Men with benign prostatic hypertrophy (an enlarged prostate) can gain help by taking selenium with vitamin E and zinc.

Selenium has also been found to reduce liver damage in people with alcoholic cirrhosis.

Selenium is also vital for the conversion of thyroid hormone to its active form (T3). The enzymes called iodothyronine deiodinases, which are responsible for the conversion of thyroxine (T4) to its active form, triiodothyronine (T3), are selenoenzymes. Selenium will help those with thyroid resistance and obesity due to underactivity of thyroid hormones.

Selenium is important for **reproduction** and both men and women may suffer with reduced **fertility** if they are selenium deficient.

Selenium deficiency is common in Australia and New Zealand where the soil content of selenium is known to be low. The fascinating article in the February 1997 issue of the *British Medical Journal,* by Margaret Rayman, brings home the problem of widespeard selenium deficiency in many European countries, Africa and China and this may be contributing to the emergence of ever increasingly virulent viruses.

In Britain all farm animals get selenium supplements because this reduces many animal diseases. It is unfortunate that humans have not caught on to the fact that selenium deficiency is a widespread and a serious problem. The recommended adult intake of selenium is 50–200 micrograms (mcg) daily, depending upon the health status of the individual. Those with excessive inflammation, skin disorders and auto-immune diseases, frequent viral infections and cancer may need higher doses. In children weighing 10–20 kilograms, a safe and adequate amount of selenium would be 50 mcg, 2–4 times weekly.

At these recommended dosage levels there are no undesirable effects from selenium.

Selenium deficiency is common and yet it is not a case of the more you take the better you will be. It is important to take the correct dose. If you overdose on selenium you can get toxic effects, such as brittle nails, garlic breath, gastrointestinal problems, hair loss, irritability, kidney dysfunction and skin eruptions. This problem of selenium toxicity is uncommon and is most often due to exposure to polluted industrial wastes. In an adult the toxic dose of selenium is around 2400–3000 mcg daily, every day for several months.

I prefer to use organic sources of selenium and the minerals boron, chromium and molybdenum, as these are better absorbed and utilised by the body. These are available in special designer yeast formulas (see page 125). I recommend one teaspoon mixed into a fresh raw fruit or vegetable juice once or twice daily. This can be taken either with food or in between meals for a quick energy boost. I myself take this powder form of immune nutrients and find that it has increased my mental and physical stamina and endurance.

Sources of selenium

This mineral can be found in meat and grains, depending upon the selenium content of the soils. The soils of New Zealand and much American farmland are low in selenium causing the food chain to also be low.

Selenium can be found in special yeasts, such as some forms of brewers yeast or designer yeasts (see page 125), kelp, brazil nuts, chicken, dairy products, broccoli, brown rice, liver, molasses, seafood, salmon, tuna, vegetables, wheatgerm, whole grains, molasses, liver, onions.

Herbs that contain selenium are chickweed, ginseng, garlic, horsetail, nettle, parsley, rose hips, uva ursi, yellow dock, yarrow, milk thistle, peppermint, alfalfa, burdock root, cayenne, fennel seed and fenugreek. One of the reasons why herbs can benefit health is that they are generally good sources of trace minerals.

VITAMIN C

Vitamin C is one of the most powerful anti-oxidants and has an especially protective effect on the inner part of the human cell. It is a great pity that humans are one of the few animal species that cannot manufacture their own vitamin C and must get it daily from the diet. Most people do not get enough, simply because they do not eat enough fresh raw food. Our ancestors living in the forests and the caves, close to fresh fruit and vegetables, berries and leaves, ingested over 2000 mg of vitamin C every day.

The daily requirement for vitamin C can vary tremendously and is increased by smoking, stress, drug abuse, excessive inflammation, allergies, infections, trauma, surgery, burns, alcohol, exposure to environmental pollutants, advancing age, chronic fatigue. The Recommended Daily Allowance (RDA) which is around 60 mg is only enough to prevent scurvy(!), and many researchers, including myself, regard this as too little for optimum health. Nobel Prize winner Linus Pauling believed that the daily dose of vitamin C should be between 2000 and 9000 mg (2–9 g) which would be too high for many people. The best available data supports a dose range of 250–1000 mg of vitamin C daily for adults and children over ten years of age. Children under ten can take 50–200 mg daily. Sometimes higher doses may be needed but should be supervised by a doctor or health practitioner.

Some people worry that vitamin C may cause kidney stones or diarrhoea; however, I have never seen this myself and most people taking vitamin C, even in large doses, need not worry about kidney stones or gout. A small number of people who are prone to kidney stones and/or gout (generally for other reasons than an excess of vitamin C) may, however, become more susceptible if they take large doses of the ascorbic acid form of vitamin C. So, to be on the safe side, persons with a past history of gout, kidney disease or stone formation should not take vitamin C without first checking with their own doctor. Generally speaking, if you drink plenty of fluids, including water, you will have no problems with vitamin C.

Many studies have shown major benefits from taking vitamin C supplements long term. Researchers from the University of California studied a large group of people over ten years, looking at the effect of dietary vitamin C. They found that women with the highest vitamin C intake had a 12 per cent reduction in death rate and men with the highest vitamin C intake had a whopping 42 per cent reduction in death rate. Those who got at least 700 mg of vitamin C supplements daily had a 60 per cent drop in death rate.

As well as being vital for recovery from chronic fatigue syndrome, Vitamin C has many other benefits, such as:

- a reduced incidence of various cancers
- a reduced incidence of asthma, allergies and viral infections (such as the flu and common cold)
- improved fertility in males
- it neutralises free radicals
- it aids the immune system to produce antibodies
- it strengthens blood vessel walls
- it helps hormonal production
- it lowers cholesterol
- it reduces stickiness of platelets and blood clots

This list is very impressive and I do hope that you are inspired by this wondrous vitamin, because there are very few things that will be able to have such a wide ranging beneficial effect in our bodies as does vitamin C.

Good food sources of vitamin C

Citrus fruit (oranges, grapefruit, lemons, limes), paw paw, strawberries, kiwi fruit, guava, mangoes, persimmons, rose hips, tomatoes, broccoli, capsicum, parsley, brussel sprouts, cauliflower, berries, green vegetables, dandelion greens.

Remember that cooking these foods destroys their vitamin C content. Thirty to 40 per cent of the diet should consist of RAW fruits and vegetables.

BIOCHEMICAL CONSIDERATIONS IN CHRONIC FATIGUE

Chronic fatigue patients have reduced cellular oxygen uptake, indicating reduced or damaged mitochondrial structure. There appears to be a blockage in the transfer of free fatty acids by carnitine into the mitochondria. Thus, there is a lack of fuel in the mitochondria. This results in a significant drop in cellular synthesis of adenosine triphosphate (ATP) the most important energy carrier in the cells (see diagram of Krebs cycle on page 8). This drop in ATP synthesis results in impairment of a number of cellular functions. In adults with severe chronic fatigue, energy production in the mitochondria may be supported with carnitine, 2000 mg daily; coenzyme Q10, 200–300 mg daily; magnesium, 1000–2000 mg daily; and taurine, 1000–2000 mg daily.

Anti-oxidants (vitamins A, C, E and selenium) have a protective effect on the mitochondria because they neutralise free radicals that are generated by normal aerobic metabolism in the mitochondria.

If viral overload is high (recurrent viral infections), it is wise to use selenium, 200 mcg daily; zinc, 50 mg daily; lysine, 1000–2000 mg daily; and, of course, B complex and vitamin C. (Reference 30.)

ENERGY HERBS

GUARANA

Tiny seeds from the fruit of this climbing shrub have been used for centuries by natives in the Amazon region of Brazil for both food and medicine. The seeds were powdered and mixed with water to make a dough-like paste and dried into chew sticks, which the Indians took to maintain energy while trekking around looking for food. Guarana is now widely used around the world, particularly in Brazil where millions of people use it every day. It is a tonic which fights fatigue, promotes alertness and aids concentration. It is best used if and when you feel tired, for a quick burst of energy and the effect lasts for several hours.

GINSENG

The ginseng root has a long history of use in Asia, where it is considered the most valuable energising herb. It is used to promote sexual energy and endurance and is considered to be anti-ageing.

GINGKO

This herb has the ability to increase blood flow in the peripheral and cerebral circulations and may increase mental energy and memory. The gingko tree is the oldest surviving tree on earth, having been around for over 200 million years. Extracts of gingko herb have been used for centuries in China, Japan and India and it is now one of Europe's most widely used medications.

STEP 3

BOOST YOUR ENERGY—CHOOSE TO HAVE A POSITIVE EXPERIENCE

Every day we are confronted with choices, indeed in this day and age there are so many experiences to stimulate the senses and intellect that selecting priorities can become a stress in itself. The greatest priority is to our mental, emotional, spiritual and physical well-being and yet, in our busy days filled with lists of things we must do, many people neglect to nuture their inner self. The inner self is always there waiting for our attention and willing and able to restore our deepest needs. As I get older I become more aware of my own need to restore my inner energy and try to set aside an hour every day to do this.

Mental and emotional stress can exert a chronic drain upon our energy and well-being. The thoughts that produce emotional turmoil are in our minds and are not always easy to control, sometimes becoming overwhelming. The greatest challenge is to become master over such negative thoughts so that they do not progress to cause emotional and physical havoc. Negative emotions can lead to the release of stress hormones such as adrenalin, while reducing the happy brain chemicals such as the endorphins, melatonin and serotonin. These chemical imbalances can lead to high blood pressure, headaches, aches and pains, spasm of the blood vessels, increased stickiness of the blood and dangerous obstructions in arteries. Yes, stress does cause a significant morbidity and mortality and shortens many lives.

In our lives, the greatest thief, which saps our being of energy and joy, is our own negative thoughts. These thoughts steal our time, flooding the moment with negativity and robbing us of enjoyment. What good is it to take the right anti-ageing supplements and follow an anti-ageing diet, if we do not enjoy the extra time these things confer upon us? Better to have a short life and a merry one too!

It is easy to protect our homes and assets from theft, with security systems and guards but it is far more difficult to protect ourselves from the mental thief within us. Especially when we think this thief is our friend and we listen to it with great respect while it tells us negative things about ourself most of the time. It is difficult to banish this part of ourselves which has probably been reinforced by society, our acquaintances, our relationships and our childhood, as it has become part of us. To banish and reject these negative thoughts and memories from the inner sanctum of our mind, we need to replace them with something else, otherwise there will be emptiness. We can replace them by concentrating upon something else, either outside of us, or within us. To do the former is easy by throwing ourselves into work, a hobby, a passion, a relationship or any number of outside activities and many people do this quite successfully. But if the negative thoughts are too powerful, they may keep creeping into our conscious minds to reduce our enjoyment and performance.

So what about concentrating on something that exists entirely within us, is singular in nature, always positive and energising and, even better, enjoyable? Have you thought of that?

An effective way to banish the mental thief is by connecting with the innate beauty and simplicity that exists in our every breath. The mental thief tells us that things are not right, we don't feel or look good, we are inferior, we are unloved, the future is uncertain, we can no longer perform, we are weak and tired, etc., whereas the inner self can make us feel good and appreciate the simple joy of being alive. After all, it is a miracle that we are alive and breathing and, even better, we are human beings.

There are techniques that can be learned to connect our conscious awareness with the internal energy that exists in us. We will be able to reject the negative thoughts and embrace the beauty and peace in every breath.What drives us crazy is our thought patterns, the negative and angry ones, that go around in circles interminably with no sense of direction and no destination. We need to get off these neuronal circuits that are so overactive that they are wearing us out mentally and physically. There will always be things to stress us out, that is life, but we can **CHOOSE** to concentrate on something else. Something positive to ride us through and hopefully bring increased understanding, acceptance and detatchment.

The Chinese have a saying, 'The birds of worry and care fly around your head, this you cannot prevent, but that they build a nest in your hair you can prevent'.

Our thoughts and emotions create an experience that we perceive as our reality—a perceived reality—but just how real and even more importantly, how enjoyable is it? Do we want to stay in it if it is not good for our mental and physical health? Sometimes we must get to the end of a road we have created with thoughts and desires, only to find that we need to start all over again with a different compass. The beginning of a new journey is always exciting and so is the journey that we take when we start to go within ourselves to renew that energy that gives us inspiration.

Here is a **breathing exercise** that may help you to achieve relaxation and better concentration. Sit in a comfortable position in a quiet place and close your eyes. Breath deeply and slowly and put your full mental concentration into your breathing. As you breath in, feel the positive energising force filling your lungs and be aware of its power. The breath of life is a gift that sustains your existence on this planet and brings the oxygen required for every cell in your body. Breathing in deeply gives you strength and power.

As you breath out fully, let all the stress and tension pass out of

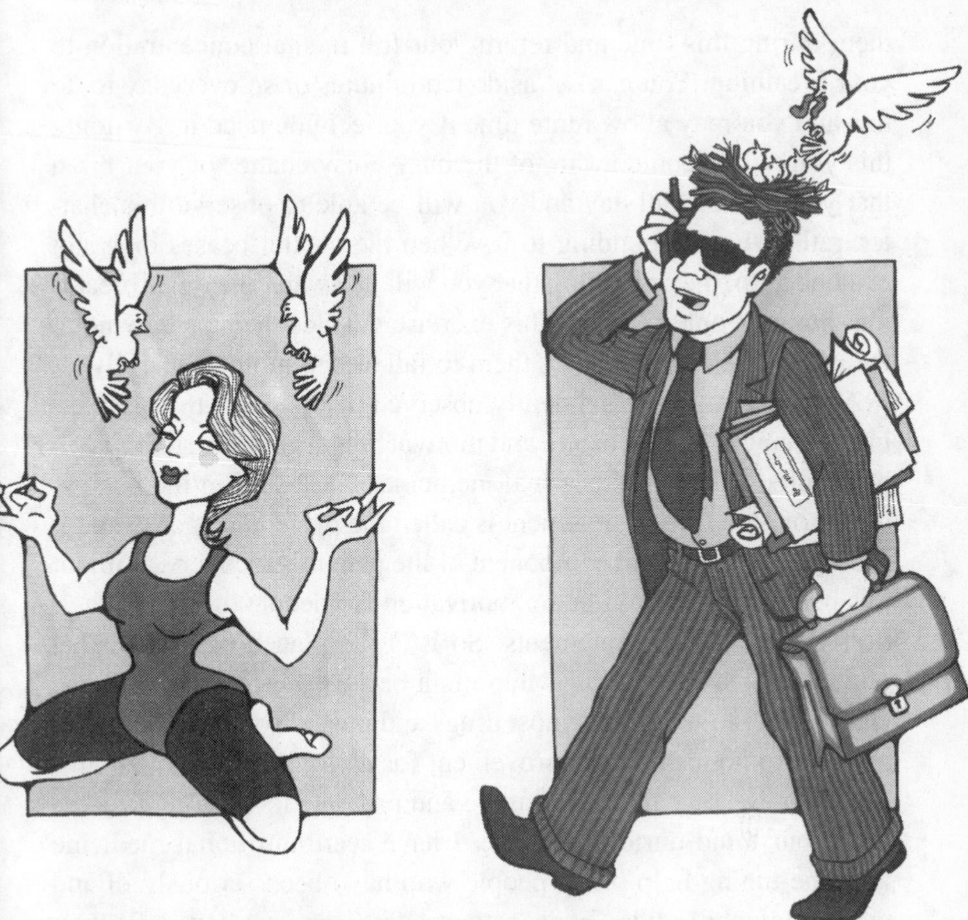

The Chinese have a saying that goes, 'That the birds of worry and care fly around your head, this you cannot prevent, but that they build a nest in your hair you can prevent.'

your body and this will make you feel peaceful. Be aware of life itself passing in and out of your body in deep rhythmical breaths. This will make you conscious of the power and beauty in your breath and the incredible fact that something so simple is keeping you alive.

If your mind tries to distract you with other thoughts, disregard them during this time and return your full mental concentration to your breathing. You can set aside ten minutes or so everyday to do this and you may allow more time if you feel you need it. By doing this you will become aware of the busy noisy chatter of your brain that you listen to all day and you will be able to observe this chatter, rather than responding to it. When the chatter ceases or is not responded to, the only thing that you will be aware of is your breathing. Some people find that this exercise enables them to unwind at the end of the day and helps them to fall asleep more peacefully.

As a doctor, I have frequently observed that people are only willing to change if I can inspire and motivate them enough, so they will have some belief in nutritional medicine. The belief in the healing power of any form of treatment is called the placebo response and it is usually a significant component of the patient's recovery. Without this belief, there would be no motivation for people to change their lifestyle and take supplements. So it is the placebo response that often works initially. This is important because nutritional medicine takes longer to work than most drugs and indeed some patients may not start to notice a big improvement for up to four or five months. So, it is necessary to hang in there and promote the healing process with your mind during this time. I have seen nutritional medicine and fine-tuning help many people who have been seriously ill and on the downhill slide. Even patients with cancer often defy their statistical prognosis with the power of nutritional medicine and Ian Gawler's book titled *You Can Conquer Cancer* and Dr Ruth Cilento's book titled *Heal Cancer*, are testimonies to these miracles that you may find worth reading.

It takes courage to turn a negative experience into a positive one and to do this you need enough self-esteem to believe in the healing force within you. Once you feel it working, it gathers momentum and things get easier.

Here is an inspiring story from one of my patients. In 1989, Ken P., a security guard from Sydney consulted me about severe ulcerative colitis, which is an inflammatory process affecting the colon. He had profuse bloody diarrhoea, weight loss and chronic abdominal pain. His brother, who was ten years older, had had the same problem and developed small bowel cancers requiring removal of his colon. Ken was using multiple anti-inflammatory drugs, which were only partially effective and gave him heartburn. His surgeon told him that he would probably follow the same path as his brother. Ken was a fairly 'macho'-type of guy and did not complain easily; however, he told me that deep down he was terrified. So, he had the motivation to change although he told me that he really did not believe that nutritional medicine was strong enough to help him. He had been under the impression that natural methods of healing were unscientific, too simple and as he told me not for 'real' men.

I gave Ken a simple program to follow because he was a bachelor and was also very busy. I told him to buy organic fruit and vegetables which he could obtain through the local health food store and to make up 40 per cent of his diet from raw fruit and vegetables. The rest of the vegetables he could cook by steaming, baking or stir-frying in vegetable stock and adding some cold-pressed virgin olive oil.

He would also buy a juice extracting machine and have two glasses of mixed raw juices daily. If these caused loose bowel actions he was to dilute them with 50 per cent water. I also told him to buy a water filter to remove all toxic chemicals from his drinking water. To supplement the fruit and vegetables he was to eat rice, beans, peas, lentils, sprouts, seafood and eggs (poached or boiled). He was to eat soy yoghurt twice daily to boost friendly bacteria in the bowel. I asked him to avoid dairy products, margarine, processed fats, land animal meats, wheat, rye, barley and oats and packaged processed foods. This is because if the bowel is severely inflamed it is best to avoid strong proteins that may be allergenic (irritating), such as gluten (found in wheat, rye, barley, oats) and cows' milk products.

I gave him a course of natural anti-inflammatory supplements, namely vitamins A, C, E and organic selenium, flaxseed oil, a multi-mineral formula and magnesium. Because he was sceptical I taught him to do the breathing exercise and after he had finished that he was to make positive affirmations to himself that he was going to become well slowly and surely.

It was two months later when I saw him again and he stated that he was only slightly better and that he missed his diet coke and hamburgers; however, he was still trying. We went through everything again and I convinced him to give it two months longer and to keep up with the positive affirmations.

Ten weeks later I saw him again and this time it was very different. He had put on weight and muscle and had a cheeky twinkle in his eyes. He grabbed my hand and shook it and gave me a big grin. He was now only on a very small dose of one drug (instead of three) and his specialist was amazed at his improvement. His bowel actions were essentially normal and he was no longer in pain. He told me that the hardest thing in his recovery had been believing that he would ever get better because his mind kept telling him negative things and dragging him down. So, for Ken, the positive affirmations had been vitally important for him to last the distance. Now that he had turned the corner I was able to enlarge his diet and reduce the dose of supplements to a maintenance level.

CHAPTER SEVEN

FIBROMYALGIA

Fibromyalgia is a common condition, especially in women over forty, and is the term used to describe pain or achiness affecting muscles, tendons and ligaments. It may be associated with joint pain and headaches and the pain is often widespread. The pain may be chronic or intermittent and to qualify for the diagnosis of fibromyalgia it must have been present for at least three months. There will be tender points in the muscles and tendons which are painful to touch and are known as 'trigger points'.

Many patients with fibromyalgia have chronic fatigue and are very sensitive to drugs and chemicals. A significant percentage of fibromyalgia sufferers have a sleep disorder because their pain does not allow them to enter the deep stages of sleep which are necessary to recharge their endocrine (hormonal) system. Another contributing factor to fibromyalgia is poor function of the mitochondria inside the muscle cells. There is insufficient production of energy from the aerobic Kreb's cycle within the mitochondria due to various blocks in the cycle (see page 8). Thus, the muscle cells must rely excessively on anaerobic metabolism to obtain energy and this leads to a build up of acidic waste products inside the muscle cell. These excessive acids, such as lactic acid and pyruvate, cause muscular inflammation and pain.

TREATMENTS

A regular exercise program is essential, although it must be built up slowly and gradually (see chapter 10).

It is important to see a physical therapist, such as a physiotherapist, massage therapist, chiropractor or osteopath before beginning your exercise program. This is because there may be problems with the joints, spine, posture or anatomical imbalances, such as a short leg or pelvic twist, that need specific treatment.

Acupuncture or specific massage techniques, such as Swedish massage or Rolfing, which is deep-tissue massage, can make a huge improvement.

NATURAL SUPPLEMENTS

These can make a big difference and combined with an exercise program can achieve cure rates of over 80 per cent. You need to take supplements to reduce inflammation in the muscle cells and to overcome the blocks in the energy cycle within the mitochondria.
To achieve this I recommend you try:

1. **Essential fatty acids**, such as flaxseed (linseed), evening primrose oil or starflower oil in a dosage of 3000–4000 mg daily. You should also boost your intake of essential fatty acids from the diet (see page 71).

2. **Vitamin E**, 500 IU, twice daily.

3. A **complete magnesium formula** containing a mixture of different types of magnesium, such as magnesium aspartate, amino acid chelate, sulphate and phosphate. Dosage varies from two to four tablets daily.

4. **Co-enzyme Q10** which is helpful for aerobic energy production in the mitochondria inside the muscle cells. Dosage varies from 30 to 200 mg daily.

5. **L-carnitine** is an amino acid (protein) that can boost aerobic

energy production in the mitochondria inside the muscle cells. Dosage varies from 500 to 2000 mg daily.

6. **Designer yeast powders** provide a broad spectrum of minerals, such as selenium, manganese, boron, molybdenum, chromium, zinc and the mitochondrial aid maleic acid (see page 125). I have found these nutrients can reduce the pain of fibromyalgia and boost muscular energy production. Dosage for fibromyalgia is two teaspoons stirred into fresh juice daily, just before food.

DRUG THERAPIES

In cases of severe fibromyalgia (FM) sufferers may be so incapacitated that they cannot sleep, hold down a job or even function at home. This may lead to depression and stress which aggravates the pain of FM and we have a vicious circle that must be broken. In such cases, anti-depressant drugs can restore sleep and reduce pain. The drug amitriptyline can be used in a dosage that varies from 5 to 200 mg daily, with smaller doses being used initially. Higher doses may cause side effects, such as drowsiness, dry mouth, blurred vision, constipation and weight gain.

These side effects can be minimised or avoided completely by starting with very small doses and gradually increasing the dosage over several weeks and by taking the total dose around 7 pm. Amitryptyline belongs to a family of anti-depressant drugs called tricyclic anti-depressants and other drugs within this family may also be tried. Although anti-depressant drugs are not habit forming or addictive, they are only available on a doctor's prescription.

Some patients with severe FM and chronic fatigue have been helped greatly by the newer generation of anti-depressant drugs known as Serotonin re-uptake inhibitors. Examples of these drugs are Prozac, Zoloft, Aropax and Effexor. These drugs are generally not sedating and are not habit forming.

Some researchers who specialise in treating patients with CFS and/or FM have found that these patients have poor function of the adrenal gland. This results in low levels of the hormone cortisone which is produced from the adrenal cortex. They have achieved good results using very small doses of cortisone (around 2.5 to 5 mg), two to three times daily. References G. A. McCain, et al., 'Diurnal Hormone Variation in Fibromyalgia Syndrome', *Journal of Rheumatology* 25 (1993) : 469–474.

I would only use low-dose cortisone in severe cases of FM and only if nutritional therapies had been tried for six months and had not helped.

I would also try non-steroidal anti-inflammatory drugs, such as Orudis or Naprosyn before trying low-dose cortisone.

CHAPTER EIGHT

FATIGUE IN SPECIAL CIRCUMSTANCES

FATIGUE AFTER HYSTERECTOMY

Seven days after the operation, begin taking supplements to speed the healing process (see fatigue after surgery page 150). If you have had a total hysterectomy where the ovaries have been removed, you may become very tired if your hormone replacement therapy is not balanced properly. Even if your ovaries have been conserved, you may still suffer with hormonal imbalances and indeed menopause may be brought on prematurely because the blood supply to the ovary has been damaged to some degree.

If you feel tired several months after your hysterectomy, have a blood test to measure the levels of the sex hormones oestrogen and testosterone and if you still have ovaries, check the progesterone level also. These blood tests will determine if you need all three hormones; namely, natural oestrogen, testosterone and progesterone. The oestrogen and testosterone can be administered in an implant in younger women or if the hormone levels are very low and menopausal symptoms are severe. Otherwise you may find that troches (lozenges) containing varying combinations of oestrogen, testosterone and progesterone are more suitable because they are weaker and the dosage is easier to control. Some women may find that conventional oestrogen tablets alone are sufficient and it takes a little trial and error before they get their hormone replacement therapy correct. Other women find that they feel exhausted and sexless after a hysterectomy unless they receive some testosterone along with the oestrogen replacement. Once again, we are all individuals and our requirements differ. I have also found that the phytoestrogen powders (see page 61) are of great benefit after a hysterectomy and prevent the hair loss that can occur after this operation. Do not be concerned that a hysterectomy will turn you into a tired old woman because in this day and age natural hormone replacement therapy and phytoestrogens can have you feeling much better that you did before the operation. Keep an eye on your hormone levels and don't become complacent. If you feel tired, ask your doctor to do a check of your blood hormone levels, say at three-monthly intervals, until you get it right.

FATIGUE AFTER CHILDBIRTH

One in three women complain of depression after childbirth and this is called postnatal depression. It is often associated with profound fatigue and many women have told me that they have never regained their energy and vitality after having a baby. This is unfortunate because with a little bit of knowledge they could be rejuvenated.

If you are depressed it is usually necessary to have an anti-depressant drug which will help enormously. You will probably need to take this for twelve months.

Many women with postnatal fatigue have lost a considerable amount of blood during childbirth and the demands of breast feeding may further deplete iron stores. It is necessary to take organic iron and spirulina everyday to help with this.

Hormonal factors must also be considered. If you are breast feeding, your ovaries will not be producing their normal amounts of sex hormones, at least while breast feeding is very frequent. So do not expect to be a femme fatale—this is normal. More significantly, in women who have lost a large amount of blood during childbirth, and especially in under-nourished women, there may be a general underactivity of many parts of the hormonal (endocrine) system. In particular, the pituitary gland and the adrenal glands may not be producing sufficient hormones, which can lead to severe fatigue. A program of nutritional supplements should boost this low hormonal state.

For postnatal fatigue I recommend:
Evening primrose oil, 4000–6000 mg daily—more if breastfeeding
Flaxseed oil, 3000 mg daily—good for breast milk and the brain
Pantothenic acid (vitamin B_5), 100 mg daily—for adrenal exhaustion
Vitamin B complex, one tablet daily—for nervous exhaustion
Vitamin E, 1000 IU daily—for adrenal and nervous exhaustion
Vitamin C, 1000 mg daily—for adrenal and immune exhaustion
L-carnitine, 500 mg daily—on an empty stomach
Magnesium, 1000 mg daily—the great relaxer
Spirulina, 2000–3000 mg daily—or iron and blood sugar problems
Selenium, 100 mcg daily—for immune exhaustion
Calcium, 1000 mg daily—for breast feeding and your bones
Also, take organic iron if you are breastfeeding, anaemic or have low iron levels—please check this with your doctor.

These are all safe to take while breastfeeding. If the baby is breast feeding and develops diarrhoea while you are on these supplements, then halve the doses.

Keep up your fluid levels with raw vegetable and fruit juices, water and teas. Many women with postnatal fatigue are chronically dehydrated which causes exhaustion, headaches and a reduced milk supply.

Some women with postnatal depression and fatigue that is slow to respond to nutritional medicine and/or anti-depressant drugs, may want to consider hormone therapy. Some studies have shown that treatment with natural sex hormones, such as progesterone, oestrogen and/or testosterone can cure postnatal depression/fatigue syndrome. While breast feeding it is possible to take natural progesterone in the form of troches or creams (see page 44). If not breast feeding, you should be able to take oestrogen and/or testosterone, probably in the form of troches and some women find that this restores their feelings of energy and happiness, as well as their sex drive. Blood tests for hormone levels may be helpful here.

FATIGUE AFTER SURGERY

This can be reduced by taking a good liver tonic (see page 111) for eight weeks which will help the liver to eliminate the anaesthetic/analgesic drugs used during the operation.

Supplements to speed up healing and reduce fatigue are:

Zinc, 50 mg daily
Vitamin E, 500–1000 IU daily
Vitamin C, 1000 mg daily
L-carnitine, 500 mg twice daily on an empty stomach
Ginseng, 1000–2000 mg daily
Kelp, 1000 mg daily
Spirulina, 2000–3000 mg daily
You may also need iron if you have lost considerable blood during the operation, so get your doctor to check this with a blood test.

FATIGUE AFTER VIRAL INFECTIONS

If you have been taking antibiotics you will probably feel more fatigued because they damage the intestinal flora and may cause candida and other unfriendly organisms to flourish in the bowel. To reduce this problem, take acidophilus yoghurt. Soy yoghurt is very good. You can also take acidophilus and bifidus powders to restore healthy flora in the intestines. These powders must remain refrigerated to retain their quality. You should also follow the energy diet or a liver-cleansing diet for eight weeks after the infection, to avoid a recurrence of the viral infection. Avoid mucous-forming foods, such as dairy products, margarines, processed foods and deep-fried foods because excessive amounts of mucous will encourage a recurrence of the infection. Make sure you eat plenty of raw fruit and vegetables. Citrus fruit is most beneficial.

If your throat is still sore, gargle with macrobiotic sea salt dissolved in warm water, twice daily after meals. You can also have steam inhalations of 3–4 drops of pure tea-tree oil dissolved in warm to hot water in a large bowl. Place a cloth over your head and breathe deeply for five minutes.

To boost the immune system take:

Vitamin C, 1000mg daily, combined with bioflavonoids such as rutin, quecertin and hesperidin.

Cod liver oil, 1000 mg twice daily, to soothe and heal mucous membranes.

Garlic, fresh cloves chopped and eaten with food are best; however, if you do not like the odour, use garlic capsules, 2000 mg three times daily with meals. Garlic is an excellent antibiotic.

Echinacea is a herb with immune-boosting properties. If your immune system is weak and you have suffered with many viral illnesses, echinacea in a dose of 1000 mg twice daily may help. Please note that those with severe allergies or auto-immune diseases should be very careful with echinacea, as in such cases the immune system is already overstimulated.

Selenium, 200 mcg daily, is of value because it is able to reduce viral replication and is also anti-inflammatory

FATIGUE AFTER TREATMENT FOR CANCER

Cancer treatments such as surgery, chemotherapy and radiation often lead to fatigue and stress. The care of cancer patients is a very specialised area and I advise them to seek out the care of a physician who has a special interest in the nutritional and naturopathic treatment of cancer patients. Such a specialist is invaluable in helping the cancer patient to restore the immune system after orthodox cancer therapies

I will suggest some general strategies to follow after treatment for cancer to rejuvenate the immune system and boost energy levels. These are:

Vitamin C, 1000 mg daily
Selenium, 200 mcg daily
Evening primrose oil, 3000 mg daily
Flaxseed oil, 2000 mg daily
Vitamin E, 500–1000 IU daily
Coenzyme Q10, 100 mg daily

According to Henry Osiecki Bsc, Grad. Dip. Nutrition & Dietetics, Coenzyme Q10 is an important therapy for many cancer patients and he recommends a high dosage of 300–400 mg daily. Henry states, 'Coenzyme Q10 has been shown to reduce tumour growth, stimulate the immune system and improve cellular energetics. It normalises cancer cell energetics, improves mitochondrial function and increases cancer cell energy production which normalises cellular function'. This is based upon the phenomena that if the mitochondrial Krebs cycle is blocked, this will cause the cell to revert to anaerobic metabolism to survive and the cell then tends to behave as a fruiting body under stress which will multiply unchecked. Thus, abnormal mitochondrial function may be related to the genesis and growth of cancer cells. To treat cancer effectively we must normalise mitochondrial function in the cells, rather than just concentrating on killing the abnormal cells. This may increase the chances of spontaneous regression of cancer (References 31, 32, 33, 34.).

Herbs that may have worthwhile immune-boosting properties are:
astragalus, echinacea, ligustrum, golden seal, pau d'arco, suma (bark, berries, leaves, roots), schizandra, garlic and mistletoe (iscador) and these should be prescribed by a doctor with special expertise in cancer treatment.

Foods that boost immunity and reduce cancer growth are: raw vegetable and fruit juices, citrus fruit, shiitake and rei-shi mushrooms, cruciferous vegetables (cabbage, brussel sprouts, kohlrabi, broccoli, cauliflower), dark green leafy vegetables, orange, yellow and red coloured fruit and vegetables, sea weeds (hijiki, wakame, kombu, arame, nori, agar-agar, dulse, kelp, Irish moss), brazil nuts, phytoestrogenic foods (see page 64).

If you have a poor appetite and/or nausea you will find the energy shakes and drinks (see pages 73 to 75) can replace a meal and are easily digested. You may also need digestive enzyme tablets or powders at the beginning of every meal.

Foods that you should reduce or avoid: foods that are high in saturated or damaged fats, e.g. margarines, deep-fried foods, butter, cheese, cream, ice cream, fatty meats, preserved meats, processed snack foods, foods that are preserved by salt-pickling, salt-curing, smoking and nitrites, foods that are charred or burnt, fats and oils that are processed, not fresh, or reheated and reused. Artificial sweeteners.

Patients who are trying to recover from cancer need the best advice and also emotional support. Dr Joachim Fluhrer MBBS, ND, FACNEM, tells us about the International Cancer Association Network (ICAN) which was formed to provide people with information regarding the choices they have to treat cancer. These are his words:

The patron of ICAN is Sir William Keys (past National President of the RSL), who successfully recovered from what was considered an incurable prostate cancer. He combined orthodox and complementary therapies and wrote a book about his journey called *Flowers in Winter*.

ICAN is associated with the German and Austrian Societies of Oncology and maintains very active contact with major cancer treatment centres around the world.

The objectives of ICAN are to:

Support freedom of informed choice in cancer treatment

Provide information on treatment options for cancer

Promote safe and effective cancer treatment

Narrow the gap between Western and wholistic medicine

Encourage and support research into complementary and effective cancer treatments

Facilitate referrals to overseas cancer clinics, if appropriate

Provide referrals for patients to complementary clinics in Australia.

At the Sydney Natural Medical Centre we provide patients with complementary cancer treatments such as nutrition, anti-oxidant therapy, immune diagnosis and therapy, Chinese medicine, recovery program after chemotherapy, surgery and radiotherapy, and we can continue treatments commenced in clinics overseas.

For more information call ICAN on (02) 9251 4140 or Sydney Natural Medical Centre (02) 9977 7888.

FATIGUE AND BLOOD SUGAR LEVELS

Unstable blood sugar levels, especially low levels (hypoglycaemia) are a common cause of fatigue. Victims of hypoglycaemia will often feel dizzy, lightheaded, nauseated, sweaty, clammy and crave sweet foods. They may have fainting spells and memory lapses.

The liver and pancreas regulate blood sugar levels and if these organs are overloaded, hypoglycaemia may occur. If you have a significant weight problem and/or a family history of diabetes you must not let hypoglycaemia get out of hand or you may increase your risk of diabetes.

Recommended supplements are:

Spirulina, 1000 mg, three times daily (can have more if needed)

Multi-mineral formula containing chromium, zinc, manganese, twice daily

Amino Acid complex, one tablet, three times daily

Livertone liver tonic, one teaspoon stirred into fresh raw juices or two capsules, twice daily before meals

Vitamin B complex, one tablet every second day, before meals

Designer yeast powder containing selenium and trace minerals, one teaspoon daily (see page 125)

Digestive enzymes, one capsule at the beginning of every meal

Many hypoglycaemics are prone to infections of candida because they are always eating highly refined carbohydrates which cause this unfriendly organism to flourish. The candida increases the cravings for sugar to ensure its own survival. If you have candida, avoid prepackaged foods containing preservatives because once these get into your gut, the preservatives are broken down and any dormant fungi in the packaged foods will start to thrive. Those with hypoglycaemia must avoid artificial sweeteners because they destabilise blood sugar levels and increase cravings for sugar.

There are many theories floating around about the correct diet to follow if you are hypoglycaemic and/or have candida infections. They differ widely and many are far too restrictive; no wonder the failure rate is high.

I suggest the following:

- Have regular meals containing complex carbohydrates (unprocessed grains, cereals, wholemeal breads and pastas, legumes, nuts, seeds)
- Have regular meals containing first-class protein (eggs, seafoods, lean fresh meat, chicken or combine three of the following four at one meal—grains, nuts, seeds, legumes)
- Eat lots of vegetables—raw and cooked
- Have unflavoured acidophilus yoghurts
- If you want something sweet, have fresh fruit, fruit sorbets, honey on a rice cake or dried fruit and nuts

I do not subscribe to the theory that hypoglycaemics need a sugar-free diet and indeed this is dangerous and will lead to severe fatigue and mental frustration and nobody ever lasts on these terribly strict diets. Provided you do not binge on large amounts of sweet foods and you are obtaining all the necessary trace minerals from the diet and the above supplement program, your body will cope with a small regular amount of sugar. Regular excercise also greatly helps to stabilise blood sugar levels. I do not agree with those who tell candida sufferers to avoid mushrooms and brewers yeasts or designer yeast powders because these things have nothing to do with candida and indeed will help to boost the immune system.

Those who suffer with hypoglycaemia/candida should avoid refined carbohydrates, such as white sugar and flour, lollies, chocolates, sweet cakes and biscuits, alcohol, caffeine and artificial sweeteners, diet colas and diet foods, processed foods containing preservatives, mouldy cheeses and foods that are not fresh.

FATIGUE AFTER EMOTIONAL STRESS OR SHOCK

This type of stress affects the nervous system which has a depressant effect upon the immune system. Try to get extra sleep and if you are not coping, get professional help from a psychiatrist or psychologist. Your fatigue may be associated with feelings of panic, depersonalisation and isolation and you may need temporary help with medication. Avoid sedative drugs and alcohol because of their addictive nature; however, if anti-depressants are required for a short time, do not worry about this as they are not habit forming. Severe depression can cause chronic fatigue and some patients find that anti-depressant drugs overcome this fatigue. Avoid excessive amounts of coffee as it may cause anxiety.

Suggested supplements are:

Vitamin B complex, one tablet daily. Some people find that intramuscular injections of B vitamins are more effective

Evening Primrose Oil, 3000 mg daily

Vitamin C, 1000 mg daily

Lecithin, 4000 mg daily

Magnesium (the great relaxer), 1000 mg twice daily

Relaxing herbs such as valerian, chamomile, hops, passionflower and hypericum can be prescribed by a herbalist. Bach flower remedies such as Rescue Remedy may help.

VEGETARIANS AND FATIGUE

If you are a strict vegan you may suffer with nutritional deficiencies that could lead to fatigue. A vegan is someone who does not eat any animal protein. In other words they strictly avoid any meats, seafoods, dairy products or other animal milks and eggs. If this applies to you and you are feeling tired and run down you may be suffering with a defiency of any of the following nutrients: **vitamin B_{12}, iron and amino acids, especially taurine.**

Taurine is found in eggs, all meats, seafoods and animal milks. If you are lacking taurine, your liver function may not be optimal which can lead to problems with bile production and fat metabolism. It is easy to take a taurine supplement and doses range from 500 to 2000 mg daily, depending upon individual needs. Those with liver problems, chemical sensitivities, allergies, epilepsy and chronic fatigue may need the higher doses.

Spirulina is a useful source of protein and iron and strict vegans may need up to 4000 mg daily of spirulina. In strict vegans, spirulina by itself is not enough and a supplement of vitamin B_{12} must be taken. If you don't like spirulina, you can buy tablets containing both iron and vitamin B_{12}. Required daily intake for vitamin B_{12} is from 5 to 50 micrograms daily and for iron is around 15 milligrams daily, and this applies for vegans as well. Blood tests to measure your levels of B_{12} and iron are important if you are a strict vegan. Iron deficiency is a very common cause of severe fatigue in premenopausal women who are menstruating regularly.

Vitamin B_{12} is a great energiser because it is essential for the production of new cells and the healthy function of the nervous system. Some people have found B_{12} tablets and/or injections very helpful for reducing allergies and food/chemical sensitivities that often accompany chronic fatigue syndrome.

Animal protein is virtually the only significant source of naturally occurring vitamin B_{12}. Even if animal protein is consumed, some people have trouble absorbing dietary vitamin B_{12} as they get older and may develop a severe B_{12} deficiency. This can be serious and lead to permanent brain damage and paralysis. In cases of severe vitamin B_{12} deficiency it is vital to receive regular injections of this vitamin.

Deficiency of vitamin B_{12} is not uncommon in vegans, especially in children or young women who go on very restricted diets. Claims that soy products (miso, tempeh, tofu, etc.), nori and other sea weeds, grains, yeast and cereals, are rich in B_{12} have been proven unfounded in several studies. You cannot rely upon these products as a source of B_{12}. If you are a tired vegan ask your doctor to measure your blood levels of vitamin B_{12} and iron and you may get a real shock. This is a simple test and most worthwhile as these deficiencies are very serious and yet so easy to remedy.

Strict vegans may also be deficient in the essential nutrient **L- carnitine** which is made in the body from the essential amino acids lysine and methionine. L-carnitine is vital for the transport of long chain fatty acids into the mitochondria which are the energy factories inside all cells. Fatty acids are the major sources for energy production in the heart and skeletal muscles. So if you are tired after exercise take L-carnitine in a dose of 500 mg twice daily on an empty stomach.

If you do not want to eat any animal products you will need to combine your food carefully to avoid deficiencies of essential amino acids. To obtain first-class protein it is necessary to combine at least three of the following four food groups at every meal—grains, nuts, seeds, legumes (beans, lentils, peas). These can be sprouted for salads if desired.

FATIGUE IN THOSE WITH HIGH BLOOD PRESSURE

High blood pressure or hypertension is, unfortunately, very common in affluent societies and greatly increases the risk of heart attacks, strokes and other vascular diseases. Many hypertensive people have to take medication to lower blood pressure and this frequently causes fatigue. The other annoying side effect of some of these medications is that they reduce sexual performance, especially in men. I have cured many patients of high blood pressure and they have been extremely grateful to regain their vitality and health. Nutritional medicine can lower blood pressure very effectively and also remove the plaque that narrows the blood vessels in hypertensives.

Firstly let us look at the things you should avoid:

1. Avoid added salt and salty foods and certain drugs. Read food labels and avoid foods that have salt, soda, sodium, MSG, baking soda or the abbreviation 'Na' on the label. Also try to avoid anti-inflammatory drugs, analgesics, over-the-counter allergy and flu remedies, diet drinks and sodas, preservatives, meat tenderisers and salty sauces such as soy sauce. Avoid supplements containing the amino acids tyrosine or phenylalanine and the artificial sweetener aspartame, which contains phenylalanine, because these amino acids can elevate blood pressure in hypertensive people.
2. Avoid saturated and damaged fats. This includes pork, sausages, bacon, ham, smoked or processed meats, organ meats, fatty meats, gravies, stock cubes, deep-fried foods, hydrogenated vegetable oils, margarine and dairy products.
3. Avoid foods containing tyramine or foods that are not fresh. This includes aged cheeses and meats, anchovies, chocolate, fava beans, pickled herrings, sour cream, sherry, wine, beer, coffee. It is best to avoid any high protein foods that have been aged, pickled or fermented.

4. Do not smoke, as this damages blood vessels in many ways.
5. Avoid excess weight, as this elevates blood pressure. The liver cleansing diet is a proven way to lose weight gradually and safely.
6. Avoid excessive stress, as this releases stress hormones which elevate blood pressure. You may need stress management or learn to meditate or try my breathing exercise on page 138. Take regular exercise as this is a proven way to reduce blood pressure and stress.

Now let's take a look at the strategies you can use to reduce blood pressure:

1. Drink plenty of fluids to help kidney and liver function. The best fluids are water, raw fresh juices (such as carrot, celery, beet, citrus fruit, spinach, watermelon, parsley, cranberry), herbal teas (such as chamomile, peppermint, dandelion, rosehips). You may sweeten with honey, if desired.
2. Increase the raw fruit and vegetable content of your diet to 40 per cent of your total food intake.
3. Increase fibre in your diet, as this will help to lower blood fat levels and thus blood pressure. Good sources of fibre are raw fruit and vegetables, grains (especially buckwheat, millet, oats and rice). Good supplemental sources of fibre are oat bran and psyllium husks and these can lower cholesterol. Make sure you take these supplemental forms of fibre at least two hours away from your vitamins and other nutritional supplements, otherwise absorption may be reduced.
4. Herbs can have a gentle blood pressure reducing effect. The best ones are chamomile, hawthorn, fennel, rosemary, valerian, hops, parsley, dandelion, chilli, and cayenne (capsicum).
5. Diversify your sources of protein. Safe sources are a combination of grains, raw unsalted nuts, seeds and legumes. If you enjoy

animal protein the best sources are fish and other seafoods, lean fresh veal or beef, skinless turkey or chicken (preferably free-range). You may have three to four eggs per week but only if they are boiled or poached (never fry them). I recommend that you should have at least three days a week where you do not eat any meat except for fish, until your blood pressure is under control.

6. Examine the quality of your sleep. Do you get adequate sleep in a well aired room? Do you snore and wake up with a choking feeling? If so, you could be suffering from 'sleep apnoea', which can elevate blood pressure and cause extreme fatigue. If you have this problem please see a doctor who specialises in sleep disorders and can investigate your sleeping pattern as this problem can be treated effectively.
7. Take supplements to lower blood pressure and reduce your risk of heart attacks and strokes. **Vitamin C** is vitally important because it protects the walls of the blood vessels and reduces their risk of rupture. Take 1000 mg daily of vitamin C with added bioflavonoids and eat foods containing vitamin C (see page 133). **Magnesium** is most worthwhile to take and indeed many hypertensives are dangerously low in magnesium, especially if they have been taking diuretic drugs. Researchers at the State University of New York found that low levels of magnesium correlated with higher blood pressure levels. They did a double blind placebo controlled study which showed that taking supplemental magnesium can result in a significant reduction in both systolic and diastolic blood pressure. This is not surprising because magnesium acts like a 'calcium blocker' thereby relaxing the smooth muscle in the walls of the arteries and lowering the pressure within them. Doses of magnesium may vary from 500 to 2000 mg daily until you achieve the desired reduction in blood pressure. Please make sure that you see your doctor regularly to assess your response.

Other useful supplements to help the blood vessels and heart are:

Garlic, fresh and/or capsules, 2000–6000 mg daily
Selenium, 100 mcg daily
L- Carnitine, 500 mg twice daily on an empty stomach
Coenzyme Q10, 50 to 100 mg daily
Essential fatty acids (evening primrose oil, flaxseed oil, olive oil), 3000–4000 mg daily
Lecithin capsules, 3000–4000 mg daily
Vitamin E, 100 IU daily. You can slowly increase this under your doctor's supervision

FATIGUE AND THE INTERNATIONAL TRAVELLER

Many business people spend their lives jet setting the globe and this stresses the body in several ways. The aircraft cabin brings together people from different countries, each one being a source of a multitude of different micro-organisms with the potential for respiratory and gut infections. The aircraft air is conditioned and recirculated so everyone on board is sharing the same air and the same airborne miro-organisms. Many such travellers come down with a new respiratory infection as well as gastrointestinal upsets. These things put an extra stress upon the immune system.

Travelling across hemispheres causes the body to go instantly from one weather season to another, often with extreme climatic changes.

Travelling from east to west or vice versa will cause time changes and this confuses the hypothalamus which controls the body's circadian rhythm based on day and night's effects. This will often lead to hormonal imbalances in the hypothalamus, pituitary and pineal glands.

To overcome these hormonal disruptions, more and more people are using the hormone melatonin which can 'reset' the clock in the hypothalamus so that you can quickly adjust to the new local time at your destination. For this purpose you need to take 3 mg of melatonin one hour before bedtime at your new destination. You will probably need to continue with this for around four to six nights when the hypothalamic clock should be fully reset. If you wake up during the night you can take another 3 mg of melatonin to lengthen sleep. The stress of repeatedly crossing time zones can be greatly reduced by the use of melatonin. For more information on melatonin, see page 18.

I also recommend taking supplements to boost the immune system with the aim of reducing your risk of contracting respiratory and gut infections. These should be taken two weeks before travel, during travel and for one week after arriving home.

The most important ones are:

1. Vitamin C, 500 mg, three times daily with food.
2. Echinacea, 1000 mg, twice daily with food.
3. Designer yeast powder, 1 teaspoonful, twice daily in juice just before food (see page 125).
4. B complex vitamins, one tablet daily with food.
5. Cod liver oil capsules, two twice daily with food.
6. Flaxseed oil capsules, 1000 mg, twice daily with food.
7. Zinc chelate, 50 mg, daily with food.

CHAPTER NINE

TOXIC CHEMICALS CAN AFFECT OUR VITAL ENERGY

This chapter was written by environmental consultant Trixie Whitmore, in collaboration with Dr Sandra Cabot

Trixie Whitmore, is the author of the best-selling books Toxic Chemical-Free Living and Recovering from ME/CFS *and* Toxic Chemical-Free Pregnancy and Child-Rearing. *She was a chemical victim who, with the help of her GP and chiropractor, rehabilitated herself by changing her lifestyle and cleaning up her environment. Her vast research into the effects of toxic chemicals clearly shows us the damage we are all suffering, from our exposure to many unecessary toxic chemicals and how this contributes to our lack of energy. In this chapter you are alerted to twentieth-century toxicity and shown simple and safe alternatives.*

Tiredness and excessive fatigue seem to be symptoms of the developed industrialised world in which we live. My own vitality and super energy disappeared after I had unwittingly experienced long-term exposure to toxic chemicals. I am now termed 'chemically sensitive' and nowadays if I am accidentally exposed, I react with fatigue which may not occur until the next day. However, I am no freak, there are many people similarly affected. In fact, everyone is being adversely affected to some degree by the toxic chemicals in our world today.

We all know that when we contract a virus or infection the immediate reaction of the body is tiredness. The body needs to rest so that the immune system can fight these invading microrganisms. Similarly, when the body absorbs toxic chemicals, it has to muster its biochemical defences to detoxify the system. Many people feel very tired after being in a smoke-filled room, or a freshly painted and/or carpeted room, for long periods of time. The toxic fumes compete with oxygen in the air so that the body gets less oxygen and a dose of toxic chemicals as well. Next time you are exposed to toxic fumes take note of any reaction.

The body reacts to toxic substances by producing free radicals which cause damage to the biological membranes on which the cells of all tissues depend for their biological functions, interfering with cellular permeability, energy metabolism and causing damage to the genetic material (Halliwell & Gutteridge, 1985). It is now generally accepted that normal ageing, as well as some diseases, are the result of gradual damage caused to mitochondrial energy production by the very small proportion of free radicals which are not terminated by the body's defence mechanisms. Alterations to mitochondrial genes (DNA) have been associated with a number of diseases, including myopathies and neuropathies. Reference: extract from a paper delivered at Toxic Chemical Load Conference, July 1993, by Dr John Pollak, semi-retired toxicologist.

Anti-oxidants can help to reduce free radical overload; however, prevention is better than cure.

It is wise and safer to rid our homes and work places of as many toxic chemicals as we can so that we can maintain our energy and minimise illness. Toxic chemicals affect our biochemistry, such as exposure to organophosphate and carbamate pesticides (insect killers) which block cellular enzymes. Their killing action works by blocking essential enzymes in the insect's nervous system. Studies are now showing that these particular pesticides, which are adaptations from the nerve gases used during the two world wars, are affecting other enzyme systems of the body. Add this to the information from Dr Pollak's paper above and it is commonsense to be aware of pesticide dangers to our health and energy levels.

An effort to clean up our environment is essential if we want our workplace, house and garden to be healthy. If we try to eliminate toxic chemicals our vitality and well-being will have a much greater chance of lasting well into old age and we will also reduce the cancers which are becoming so common in today's world.

'What a lot of nonsense', you might say. 'I'm feeling fine! I have my house and office sprayed regularly for pests and it does not affect me. And I use strong solvents and cleaning chemicals in the bathroom and kitchen as well as spraying the garden regularly for pests'. Think about it. You may not have any visible effect now, or maybe you have felt tired after being exposed to such chemicals but they do catch up with us all at some stage. I have seen small children affected adversely by toxic chemicals. Recently, a young boy who was an acqaintance of mine spent over two weeks in bed and could not lift his head or limbs after exposure to a floor stripper in a toy shop which contained a 30 per cent concentration of the chemical 2-butoxyethanol. This was confirmed by his doctor who is knowledgable in environmental illnesses.

Beware of chemicals called xenoestrogens which have a similar chemical structure to human oestrogen and can mimic the effect of our own natural oestrogens, disrupting the balance of hormones in our bodies. Xenoestrogens are environmental pollutants which are ubiquitous in our food, air and water supply, being found in things like plastics and pesticides. They get into our bodies via the food chain and lodge in fat cells, particularly in the reproductive organs, breast tissue, brain, liver and hormonal glands. They may increase our risk of cancer in these areas of our body.

In these days of clever advertising we have unwittingly become 'chemical victims' as well as polluters. We are told that our houses and offices will not be clean unless we use chemical cleaning and disinfecting products and pesticides. Every insect is a potential danger to be eradicated. The only people who really benefit are those who make and sell the myriad of products on the shelves. Rather than support the manufacturers of toxic products, let's discriminate and support those who are caring for us and our environment. There are safer alternatives based on natural ingredients. Read the labels. Many health food stores sell organically based cleaning products.

Products and items which should be avoided:

Strongly perfumed petrochemical-based cosmetics, toiletries and shampoos.
Solvent-based cleaning products and polishes.
Pesticide treatments of houses and offices.
Freshly carpeted and painted premises—allow outgassing by heating and airing before occupation.
Disturbance of leaded paints.
Disinfectants containing phenol.
Lindane or malathion head lice treatments.
Dichlorvos pest strips.
Pesticides and fungicides in the garden.

'How can I live without these things?', you ask. 'Very easily', I answer. After all, our grandparents kept the house clean with laundry soap, bi-carbonate of soda, vinegar and lavender to deter pests. They used vinegar and sugar to preserve food.

I had to change my lifestyle twelve years ago and now I never think twice about it. Interestingly, many of the chemicals which made me ill are now on the International Agency for Research on Cancer of the World Health Organisation (IARC) carcinogen list.

Here is a list of some non-toxic alternatives which you may find useful.

GENERAL CLEANING

Use bi-carb and laundry soap. Moisten sponge, rub with soap, sprinkle bi-carb liberally as you would a powdered cleanser. This will form a paste which will clean any surface.

MOULD

Sprinkle bi-carb onto tiles, spray with vinegar (it will froth), leave overnight. Scrub and rinse. Salt and lemon juice kills mould, as does tea-tree oil.

REFRIGERATOR AND OVEN

Wipe out the fridge with bi-carb and water. Rinse well, add a little vanilla. For oven, make a thick paste of bi-carb and water, coat a sponge liberally with this paste and apply to oven surfaces, warm oven and wipe clean. Recoat with a thin paste of bi-carb and water and leave on while cooking. This forms a barrier and makes the next clean much easier.

PAINTWORK

Laundry soap and water plus some elbow grease seems better than detergent.

DISHES

A detergent based on coconut oil, rather than benzene, is preferable. Soap and water, together with bi-carb for grease is just as good. Always wear rubber gloves when cleaning as all soap and detergent products will dry the natural skin oils.

LAUNDRY

Pure soap powder (no perfume) or organically based laundry liquid. Add a few drops of pure tea-tree oil to eradicate bacteria from the laundry water before you turn the washing machine on. Eucalyptus oil applied to greasy stains before washing will remove them. A few drops of eucalyptus, tea-tree oil or lavender oil will nourish and protect woollens.

DISINFECTANT

Tea-tree oil or a few drops of iodine.

POLISH

Furniture polish can be made from beeswax and lemon oil.

PESTS THAT ANNOY HUMANS

Place borax and honey 50/50 on an ant trail but keep away from children and pets. Talcum powder will also deter ants.

For cockroaches, sprinkle borax behind appliances out of the reach of children or place receptacles with greased sides in the cupboard.

Fill the bottom of the receptacles with wine and brown sugar or pet food. The cockroaches will climb into the receptacle and die with their eggs. Similarly, sticky (non-toxic) traps, available from health food stores, will stick cockroaches and eggs together for disposal. Plaster of Paris and icing sugar will solidify in their gut; however, they may lay their eggs before dying and continue the cycle. Protect clothes in cupboards from moths and silverfish with citronella, lavender or eucalyptus. Deter flies with citronella or lavender and buy a fly swat, it makes for good sport and extra exercise! Fly traps can be made from plastic bottles with small 2.5 cm square holes punched in the side. Quarter fill the bottle with a mixture of vanilla, water and Vegemite.

To deter mosquitoes, rub yourself with fresh mint or citronella and sleep under a mosquito net.

PESTS THAT ANNOY PETS

There are herbal dog and cat products available. Brewers yeast is great for fleas and you can brush it into the fur and sprinkle one teaspoon daily onto their food.

PESTS IN THE GARDEN

Wood ash sprinkled on leaves will take care of moulds. Newspaper laid between rows will entice snails and slugs to hide during the day. It is then easy to remove them onto the grass for the birds to eat. For affected indoor plant leaves, sprinkle pepper onto damp leaves or spray with a mixture of chilli, water and mild detergent. Garlic spray will deter many pests.

For more information refer to the books *Toxic Chemical-Free Living and Recovering from ME/CFS* and *Toxic Chemical-Free Pregnancy and Child-Rearing,* available from PO Box 266, Pymble, 2073.

CHAPTER TEN

EXERCISE FOR FITNESS

EXERCISE FOR LONGEVITY AND ENERGY

Some say *'I am in shape'*
Some say *'I am out of shape'*
Some say *'The shape I am in'*
Some say *'The shape of things to come'*

I SAY *shape up or ship out, You can't be 'in' shape if you're out and if you're out how do you get in? You get in by going out and shaping up!* (Bob Cooper)

GETTING ON

'Getting on' is a familiar saying we've all heard and perhaps said at one time. What kind of mental picture do we have when we think of 'getting on'. The face looking more mature, a few wrinkles here and there, feeling less energetic, the posture not as straight and strong as it should be. Feeling more comfortable being less active. Losing the urgency for dynamic movement. These are just the natural tendencies of the ageing process. There's nothing wrong with it, it's just part of us. But as we are getting older we need to remember that our body is a moving machine, specifically designed for functional, dynamic action. Therefore 'getting on' doesn't mean giving up.

Given that you are basically a healthy person you can make your 'getting on' years exciting and stimulating. How? With a little knowledge and a lot of enthusiasm you can have the choice of slowing that wonderful 'thing' called the ageing process. You will discover within these next few pages exercises, techniques and programs that are easy to understand and follow and are fun to do.

TO MOVE OR NOT TO MOVE?

Through passionate dynamic movement we were conceived. We came into this world kicking and screaming. As we grew we learned to sit, crawl, walk, run, jump and leap. Our school yard games were energetic and exhilarating, leaving us breathless and full of energy. As we grew into young adults our dynamic activities were more specific and we began to quieten down a little. As we matured, our activities were somewhat governed by our position in the workplace. However, we were still forced to be energetic.

In bygone days, lawns were mowed manually, using body energies. The floors were scrubbed and polished by hand and even the good old washing machine needed some manual assistance. Children were pushed in prams and strollers with wheels that worked! Slowly and surely things have changed. The age of automation arrived and whenever we can we press a button, switch on a power point, take a lift or ride up an escalator, hop on a bus or train and drive our cars. We sit at computers and watch television and move as little as possible.

NATURAL AGEING

As we get older there's a tendency for natural ageing to occur in some of the structures and functions in our body. These we need to accept as part of 'getting on'. We can take action to slow the ageing process in our bodies by maintaining a positive attitude to cope with life's little challenges, especially as far as our body is concerned. As we have the power to control our bodies, let's see what we can do to hold back the ageing process. We can achieve this by increasing our daily dynamic activities and doing specific exercises that will improve our aerobic power, heart/lung capacity, endurance, strength, muscle tone and flexibility, all of which allow us to look and feel good.

Before we go on to explore the variety of activities suitable to longevity, let's take a good look at how we hold ourselves upright.

POSTURE

You may have been told as a child to 'stand up straight; pull your shoulders back'. Posture refers to how we hold our body. It is influenced by our height, personality, heredity, occupation and emotions. Poor posture at any age is not attractive and in a middle-aged person can make you look much older than you really are. To check your posture you need to be aware of your habitual movements. Are you stooping over, slouching, dropping your shoulders forward and allowing your head to protrude? Sagging stomach muscles and slouching shoulders, which pull the head and neck forward, place a stress on the lower back and put pressure on the nerves and discs along the spine.

Consider your body to be made up of building blocks all nicely placed on top of each other. When one of the building blocks comes out of line the rest of the structure suffers. This example can be applied to our skeletal structure. If the muscles that hold our body upright are not in balance, i.e. one section is too weak or too strong, our bones will be pulled in different directions causing bad posture, stressing our joints and body. We can correct this by becoming aware of how we walk, stand and sit. Try this little exercise!

Standing with your feet flat (without shoes), allow your hips to balance on your legs distributing your weight evenly over your feet. Vacuuming your diaphragm close to your spine, imagine yourself growing very tall. Lift your ribs away from your waist, expanding the chest and back and relaxing the shoulders. Gently get the feeling of stretching upwards. You may have a tendency to hold your breath. Concentrate on breathing rhythmically. With practice, this feeling of good posture will become second nature.

Through awareness and muscle control a well aligned body looks attractive, feels buoyant and uses energy efficiently.

HOW TO HELP SLOW THE AGEING PROCESS

Most of us are aware that fitness is important, that being fit is good for you. So, what is fitness? Basically, physical fitness is having the energy to perform your daily activities with enough energy left at the end of the day to enjoy your leisure time. To improve fitness for health and longevity we need to consider the following five areas:

* Cardiovascular fitness
* Muscular endurance
* Muscular strength
* Body fatness
* Flexibility

Cardiovascular fitness is the ability of the heart and lungs to supply the body with oxygen needed to convert food into energy. It also reduces the risk of coronary heart disease.
Muscular endurance is the ability of the muscles to work continuously with less fatigue. It also improves muscle tone.
Muscular strength helps protect the joints from injuries and allows daily activities to be performed without undue strain on the muscles.
Body fatness (composition) means a certain level of body fat is important, not only for appearance but also to help reduce the risk of heart disease, cancer and high blood pressure.
Flexibility helps prevent postural defects and back problems in later life due to lack of muscle elasticity. Regular stretching improves flexibility.

The most effective type of long-term exercise is **aerobic exercise.** Aerobic means 'with air'. That is, breathing in air and oxygen continually to supply oxygen to the working muscles. The activity needs to be continuous at an intensity that suits your fitness level. To ensure the exercise is, in fact, aerobic, remember the word FITT.

Frequency: at least three times a week, five times is better.
Intensity: exercise at 65–75 per cent of your maximum heart rate*.
Time: twenty minutes CONTINUOUS is the minimum, 30–60 minutes is better.
Type: type of exercise, aerobic classes, running, swimming, cycling, brisk walking, cross-country skiing, any activity that makes you huff and puff, and your heart beat strongly.

* Maximum heart rate is calculated by subtracting your age from 220.

With aerobic exercise the heart and lungs become stronger, which lessens the risk of heart disease. Fat particles may clog the inner walls of the arteries leading to the heart with the possible result being a heart attack. In aerobic exercise the blood rushes through the arteries at speed, carrying away fatty particles for elimination.

Aerobic exercise is an excellent way to lose body fat. When exercise begins, the body uses its muscle glycogen (muscle food) stores first, keeping fat as a reserve fuel. After twenty minutes the muscle food has been used so the body has no choice but to draw on its stores of body fat for energy. Hence, the importance of doing continuous aerobic exercise for MORE than twenty minutes.

A good way to get aerobically fit is to attend aerobic classes. They keep you motivated while improving your strength and endurance.

IF YOU DON'T USE IT YOU LOSE IT

Muscles need to be used! They need to be contracted to keep them strong, toned and healthy. When we use our muscles they become firm and shapely. When we don't use our muscles they become soft and flabby.

Let's take a look at toning and shaping. You may be familiar with abdominal exercises, push-ups, squats and knee bends. These are basic exercises that can use our own body weight to be effective. Another way of toning and shaping our body is through resistance training whereby we contract our muscles against a variable resistance. That is, we can use free weights as in weight or resistance training. This kind of muscle shaping is very effective and good results can be obtain in as short a period as six weeks. Especially if the training is well programmed and monitored. Correct training can be done by people of any age—even if you're ninety.

Resistance training does not actually burn off body fat as in aerobic exercise but it does help food to be used for energy. It is a preconceived idea that stomach exercises will slim your stomach; in fact they will tighten and tone the muscles, but if you have fat on top of the muscles, you will have to do aerobic work to get rid of the fat. Circuit training is a very effective way of increasing your aerobic capacity and toning the muscles as the circuit is a combination of resistance work and aerobic exercise. Circuit training is best done by joining a specific venue offering circuits as part of the overall service.

THE BENEFITS OF MUSCLE TRAINING

1. Muscle training tones and strengthens muscles to improve appearance and make clothes look better.
2. Stronger muscles help protect joints against instability and injury.
3. If stretching is carried out before and after exercise, postural defects, due to poor strength and flexibility, are improved.

4. Muscle training improves muscular endurance allowing muscles to work for daily activity.
5. Working through a full range of motion increases your flexibility, improves your mental functioning and also increases bone density which in turn may prevent osteoporosis.
6. Muscles metabolise more internal energy when they are toned.

Some exercises are able to be learned from books, by reading the text and practising the skills. Some of them you can learn from videos but as far as circuit or resistance training goes, it is best to visit a venue where there are qualified instructors to assist you. This will ensure that your exercise routines are both safe and effective.

SOFT EXERCISES

Stretching allows us to become more aware of our body's system of muscles, bones and joints. Stiffness is a lack of suppleness or mobility and gradual stiffness is part of the ageing process. This process can be slowed by regular stretching.

Stretching releases tension in the muscles, eliminating lactic acid and decreasing muscle tightness after exercise, bringing in nutrients and improving the blood supply to the muscles. It also assists in the co-ordination between muscle groups, improving posture. Muscles and joints are very dependant on each other. If a muscle is tight it inhibits movement of the joint and if the joint is stiff the muscle is unable to contract to its full capacity.

Stretching is an effective way of refreshing a tired body and aids relaxation.

A fit healthy body has strength and stamina, suppleness and stability. Hard exercise develops strength and stamina while soft exercise develops suppleness and stability...(Arthur Balaskas and John Stirk, Soft Exercise The Complete Book of Stretching).

FOR MAXIMUM LONGEVITY IT IS IMPORTANT, IF NOT IMPERATIVE, THAT WE PERFORM THE TYPE OF EXERCISES MENTIONED (AEROBIC ENDURANCE, RESISTANCE TRAINING, FLEXIBILITY AND RELAXATION TECHNIQUES.)

ANOTHER EXERCISE OF IMPORTANCE

Although all exercise is important to the body, of special importance to both men and women is the pelvic floor exercise.

In women, the pelvic floor contains the bladder and its outlet, the vagina, the womb and the rectum. The pelvic floor supports these important body parts, keeping them tucked up inside the pelvis. The pelvic floor muscles rely on their tightness and strength to keep the bladder and back passage under control. These muscles have a hard job to do because gravity pulls **everything** downwards.

As we get older, the muscles stretch and find it harder to do their job. Putting on weight, coughing a lot or carrying a baby inside you for nine months, puts a lot of extra strain on the pelvic floor muscles. When these muscles are strained too much they gradually become weak and are unable to work as well as they used to. Instead of everything being tucked up in your pelvis, things can sag downwards. A prolapsed uterus means that the womb is sagging down into the vagina, the other parts can sag too. Incontinence is another problem caused by weak pelvic floor muscles. Research has shown that 30–40 per cent of women have weak pelvic floor muscles. So what can be done? Again we have the control through exercise.

HOW TO EXERCISE THE PELVIC FLOOR MUSCLES

Sitting comfortably on a chair with knees apart at first, 'close the lift doors' by squeezing together the muscles around the edge of the vagina. Squeeze harder and further, taking the lift up to the first floor. Bring the lift back to the ground floor and then open the doors again by relaxing the muscles. See how many times you can squeeze the muscles before they become tired. The longer you can hold the pelvic floor contraction the stronger the muscles will become.

This exercise should be performed on a daily basis and as often as possible.

In men, the pelvic floor supports the rectum. Through the action of the hips and buttocks during sexual intercourse, the anal passage usually remains tight and strong. However, with the decrease in sexual activity because of 'getting on' there is a real possibility of anal prolapse. The exercise for the pelvic floor in men is a similar feeling as for the women's exercise only this time only the buttocks are used. An easy and effective way of doing this is to lie on the back with feet on the floor and knees bent. Keeping the lower back close to the floor and tilting the hips, squeeze the buttocks and vacuum them to the naval. Squeeze, hold for a few seconds then release. Repeat the exercise until muscles begin to tire.

The pelvic floor exercises are very important as a preventive measure against possible surgery, especially as we are 'getting on'.

Let us now review the qualities of fitness and the effect of it on the ageing process.

USE IT OR LOSE IT

The heart:

Fit—strengthened, circulates more blood per beat, with a lower resting heart rate.

Unfit—weakened, circulates less blood per beat with a higher resting heart rate.

Blood vessels:

Fit—larger, more elastic, freer circulation and lower blood pressure.

Unfit—constricted, inelastic, clogged with fat and elevated blood pressure.

Lungs

Fit—expanded capacity for oxygen absorption and waste expulsion.

Unfit—restricted capacity for oxygen absorption and waste expulsion.

Metabolic rate:

Fit—internal energy increased. More calories used in all activities and promotes leanness.

Unfit—lower metabolic rate and less calories consumed per activity, leading to accumulation of more body fat.

Body composition:

Fit—lean with less fat and more muscle mass and bone.

Unfit—more fat with less muscle and bone.

Bones:

Fit—stronger, more dense and resilient.

Unfit—weaker, more porous and brittle.

Joints:

Fit—able to work through a greater range of movement.

Unfit—stiff and restricted.

Muscles:

Fit—stronger, firmer, more defined and efficient. Tending to burn more calories.

Unfit—weaker, less tone and less efficient. Burning fewer calories.

Mental functioning:

Fit—alert, more clear and concentrated, with less boredom and fatigue.

Unfit—fatigued and bored, dull, worried and distracted.

Emotional functioning:

Fit—more patient, tolerant, relaxed and enthusiastic.

Unfit—impatient, critical, tense and depressed.

Self-concept:

Fit—more confident with positive appreciation of self.

Unfit—less certain, more doubtful and self-conscious.

Health risks:

Fit—healthier heart, lungs, blood vessels, liver, bones and body composition.

Unfit—increased risk of heart and lung disease, diabetes and broken bones.

Quality of life:

Fit—more active, greater vitality and endurance leading to longevity.

Unfit—inactive, generating less vitality and endurance, tending towards illness.

These are the basic components to fitness and longevity. Exercising with consistent effort will certainly slow down the ageing process.

SOMETHING ABOUT FITNESS CENTRES

People often begin a fitness program with good intentions, only to find that after a few weeks they lack the motivation and inspiration to continue. This lack of self-motivation and perseverance leads to feelings of inadequacy, hopelessness and failure. This feeling of low self-esteem does not encourage energetic movement and so we have a Catch 22 situation. No exercise because you feel bad and you feel bad because you don't exercise.

Attending a fitness centre or a sports club that has gym facilities helps to increase your motivation and keep you on track with your fitness program. However, for some people, the idea of attending a fitness centre can be very off-putting. Mainly due to three preconceived ideas:

(a) That they have to be fit and thin before they go.
(b) That they have to be young.
(c) That they have to be trendy.

None of the foregoing is true.

Unfortunately some fitness centres do not effectively market towards 'grey power' (the ones that are 'getting on'). That of course does not mean that you're not welcome in the gym. Therefore, it's up to you to make the first move. Take a deep breath, walk through the gym doors (you are allowed to wear track suit or T-shirt) and ask the reception staff for HELP! You will be surprised by the welcome and service you'll receive, not to mention the added benefits that such a venue could offer, e.g. fitness assessments, graded aerobic classes which will include low impact, step, toning and stretch classes. Computerised equipment for strength and cardiovascular fitness are fun to use and can take the boredom out of exercise.

An added benefit of attending a centre is the friends you'll make through the common effort of getting fit.

Come out of your comfort zone, make an effort and walk through that door!

If a fitness centre or club is not your 'cup of tea', remember that some exercise is better than none and as the name of the game is moving. Consider activities such as tennis, swimming, cycling, walking, dancing, yoga, etc. At the moment, personal training is very popular. A good personal trainer will set programs especially to suit your lifestyle and needs, ensuring that you stay motivated and on track. However, a tailor-made fitness program with supervised activities, as in a fitness centre, will produce fast, positive results at a reasonable price. 'Stickability' is what it's all about.

In the following pages, we will give you some specific exercises that tone and strengthen all the muscles. We suggest you do a total of thirty minutes exercise daily. Start with five minutes daily, gradually building up to thirty minutes daily, over a four-week period. If you suffer with any musculo-skeleton problems you should consult a physiotherapist before doing any of these exercises.

Stretching

The aim of these stretching exercises is to improve flexibility and promote relaxation by stretching of the major muscle groups.

Remember to keep your breathing soft and rythmic and with every outward breath relax your body more and more. Over-stretching causes the muscles to shake, so relax the stretch and start again. If a position is painful to you, don't do that particular stretch. Each stretch should be held between 10 and 20 seconds. Take your time and enjoy! Follow the diagrams carefully.

Back extensors

Curl into a ball.

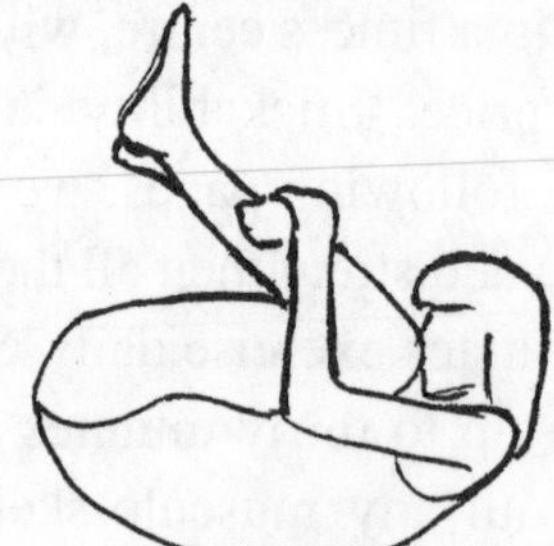

Quadriceps

Hold you left foot with your right hand and vice versa using the free hand to balance if necessary.

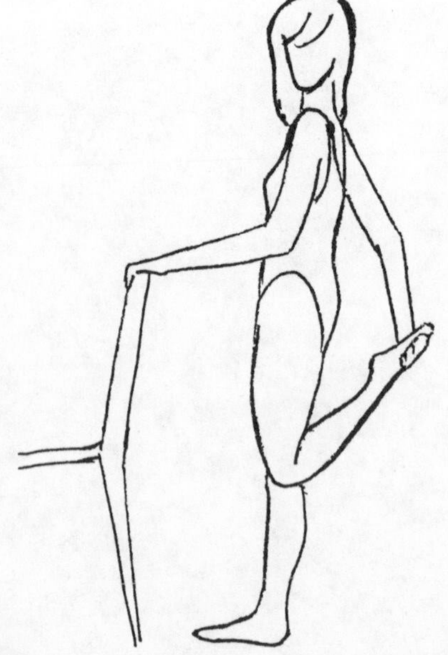

Buttock Stretches

Keep both buttocks on the ground with your back straight.

Press against your knee as shown while turning your leg away from your body.

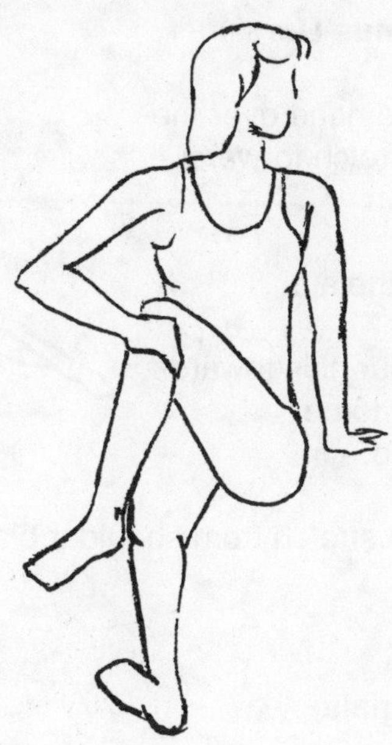

Hamstrings

Keep your lower back pressed to the floor.

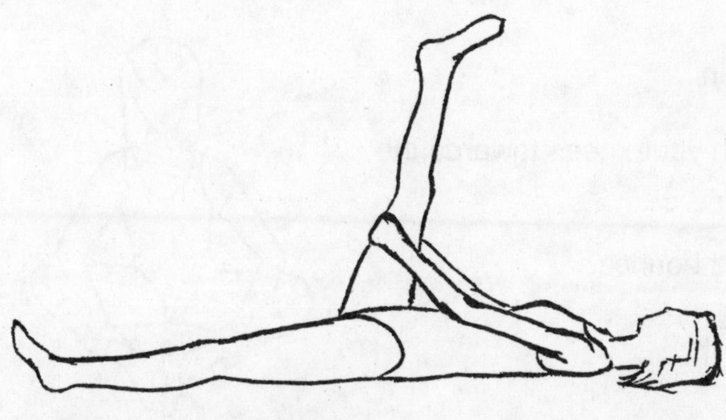

Latissimus Dorsi

With one hand over the other, stretch forward as shown.

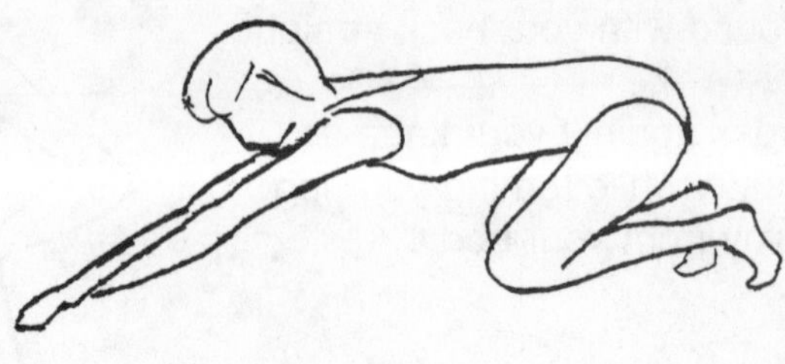

Hips in the air.

Lean your hips towards the side to be stretched.

Feel the stretch from shoulder blade to armpit.

Abdominals

Hips remain on the floor.

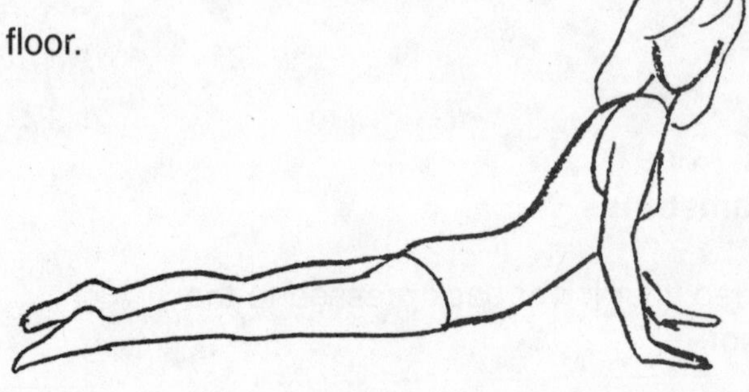

Groin

Push your knees towards the floor.

Don't bounce.

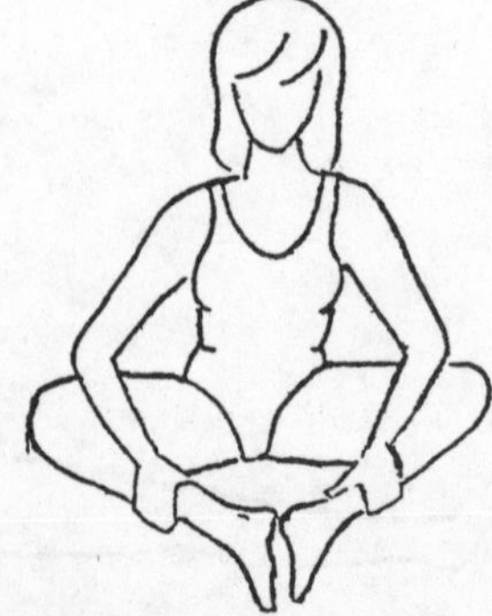

Neck

Gently pull your chin to your chest

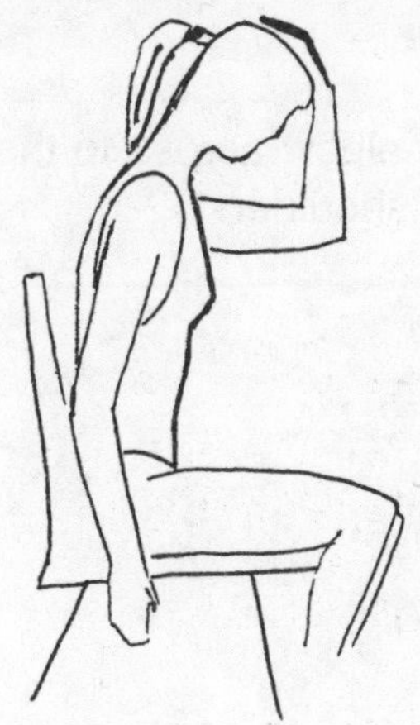

Pull your ear to your shoulder

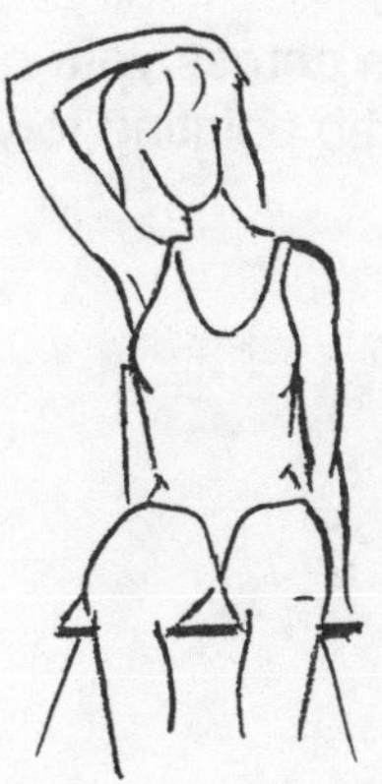

With your right hand on your head, quarter-turn it to the opposite shoulder and vice versa.

Pull your chin to your chest.

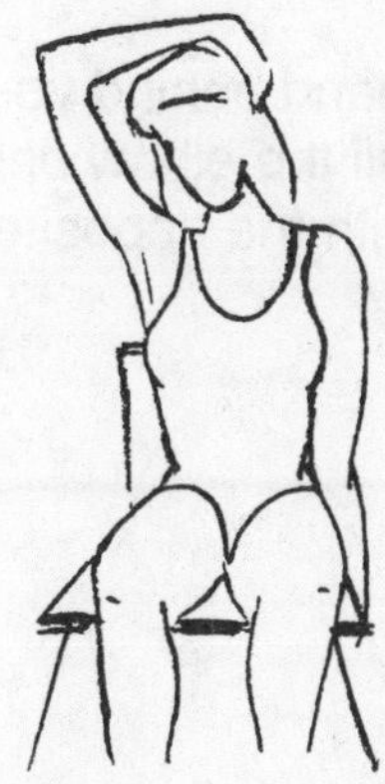

Shoulder

Pull your elbow across to the opposite shoulder.

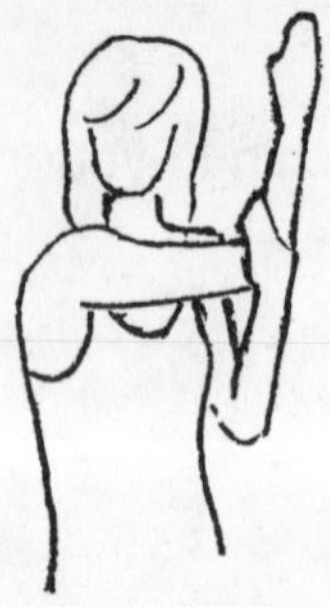

Hold your arm across your body with your thumb pointing towards the ground.

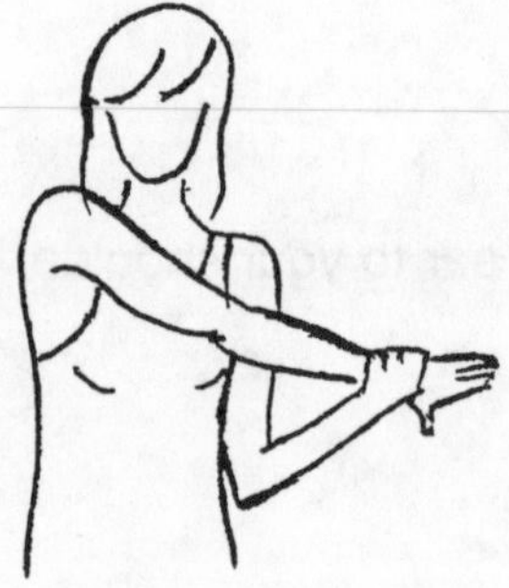

Triceps

Place your hand behind your head and pull the elbow behind your head with the opposite hand.

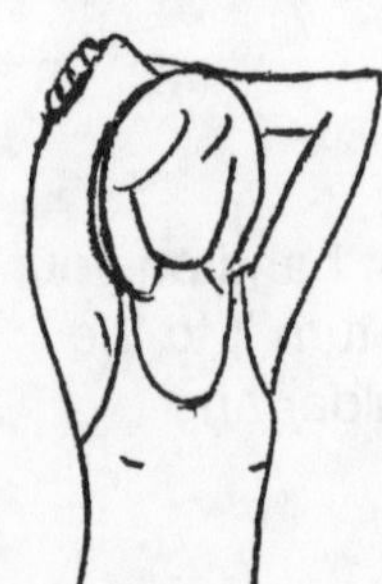

Biceps

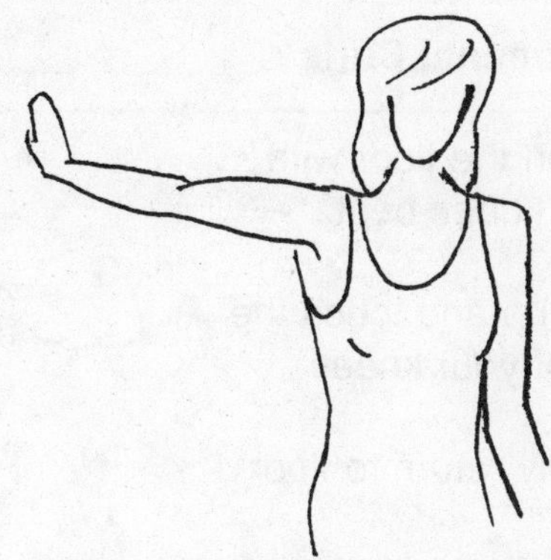

Hold onto a door at arm's length with your thumbs down.

Turn your body away from the arm and let your shoulder roll in.

Pectorals

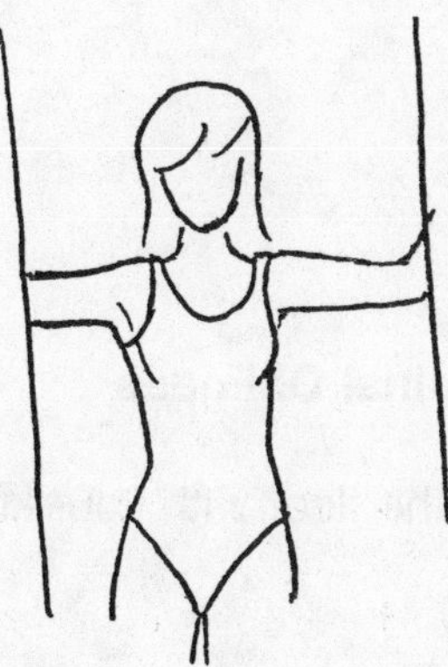

Place your elbows against a doorway and lean your body forwards.

Exercises

Abdominal Curls

Lie on the floor with your knees bent

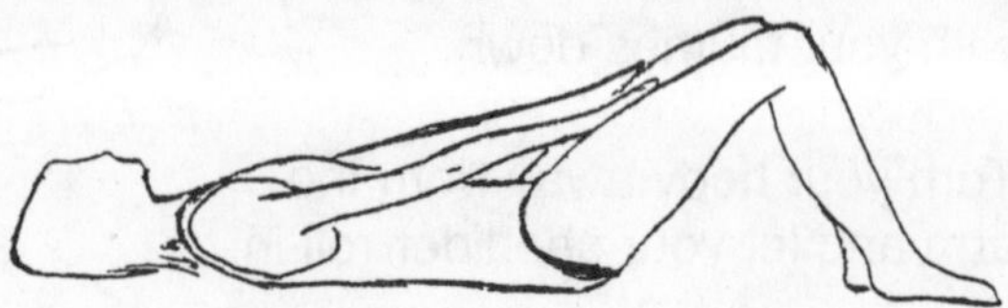

Curl up and touch the top of your knees

Slowly return to floor

Do not throw your head and shoulders up, pull with your abdominals

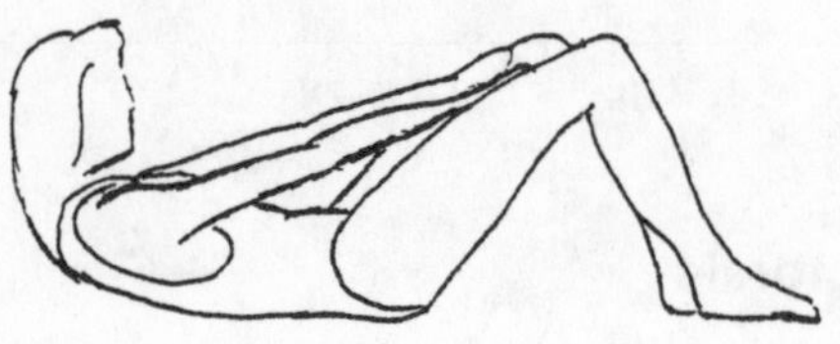

Abdominal Obliques

Lie on the floor with your knees bent

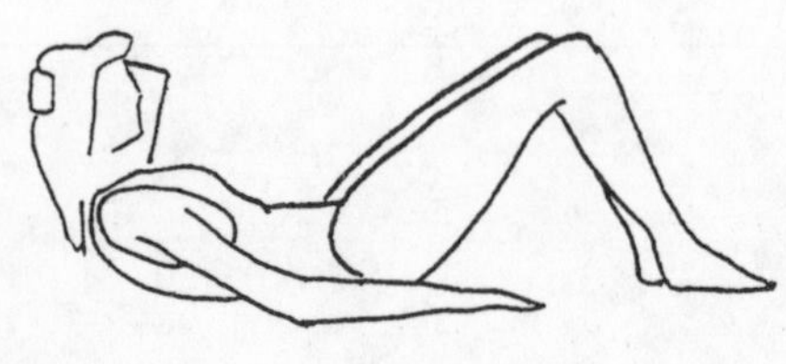

Place one hand on the floor next to your body and the other hand behind your head

Slightly raise your head off the ground and move the elbow of the hand behind your head towards your hip

Lower Abdominal Tucks

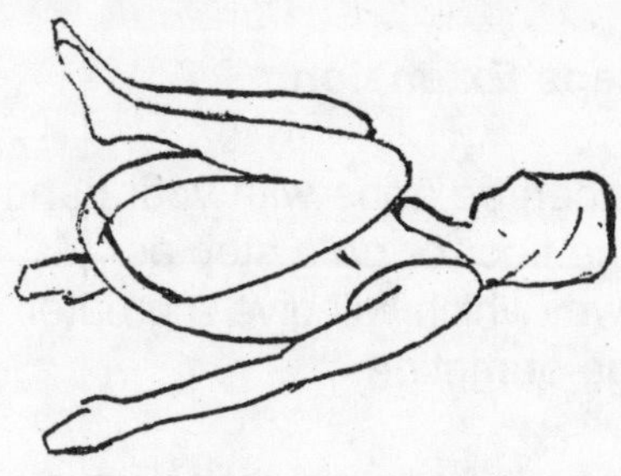

Keep your lower back pressed to the floor.

Lie on your back and place your arms on the floor next to your body with the palms down.

Bend your knees with your feet close to your buttocks.

Pull with your lower abdominals, rolling your knees to your chest and lift your buttocks off the floor.

Hip Lifts

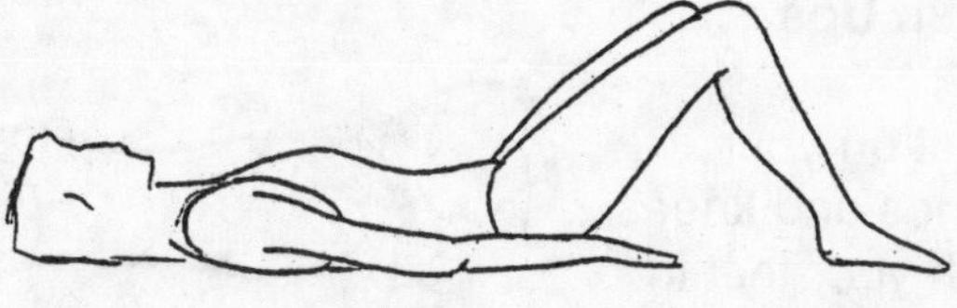

Lie on the floor with your arms next to your body with the palms down.

Squeeze your buttocks and inner thighs.

Slightly lift your buttocks and the lower part of your back while clenching your buttocks.

Rotate your pelvis upward. Do not lift your back and rest on your shoulders.

Triceps Extension

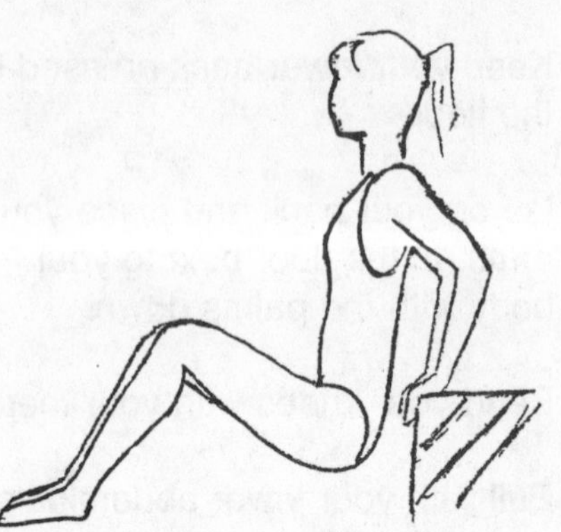

This can be done with your hands on the floor or on a step as shown, which will give a greater range of motion.

Rest your body weight on your arms not legs.

Press up and down bending your elbows. Keep elbows slightly bent in the top position

Push Ups

Rest on your hands and knees with your feet in the air as shown.

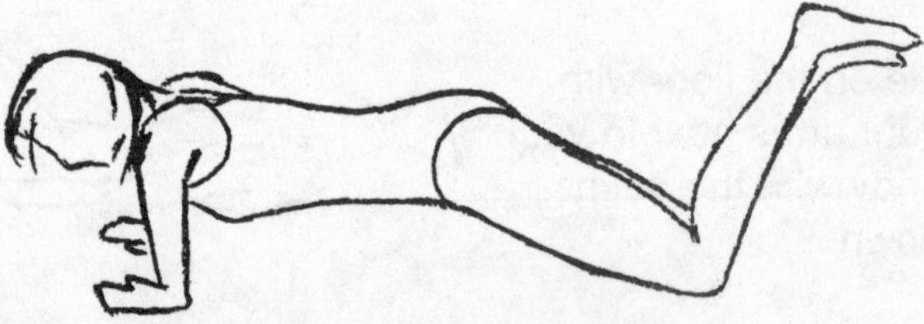

Keep your body in a straight line throughout the movement with your hands placed 10–15 cm wider than your shoulders.

Keep your head up and lower yourself to the floor. Don't lie down and don't leave your hips in the air.

Press up to the starting position but do not lock elbows.

Back Extension

Lie face down on the floor with your hands behind your head and your elbows up.

Lift your torso off the floor and squeeze your buttocks.

Lower your body slowly.

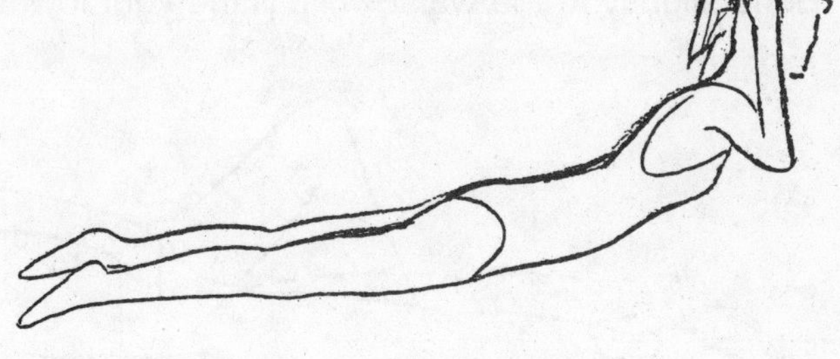

Side Leg Raises

Lie on your side as shown, lifting your top leg to about 45˚ and lower it down again.

Flex your foot, i.e. pull your toes towards your shin, turn your foot down with your big toe towards the floor.

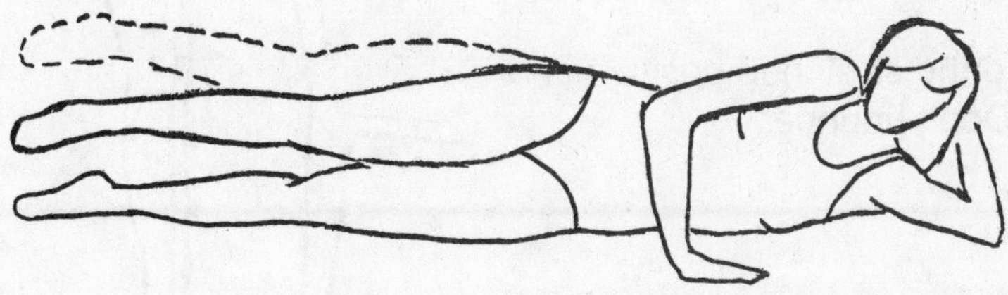

Inner Leg Lifts

Lie on the floor as shown.

Bend slightly at the waist while lifting your lower leg up and down.

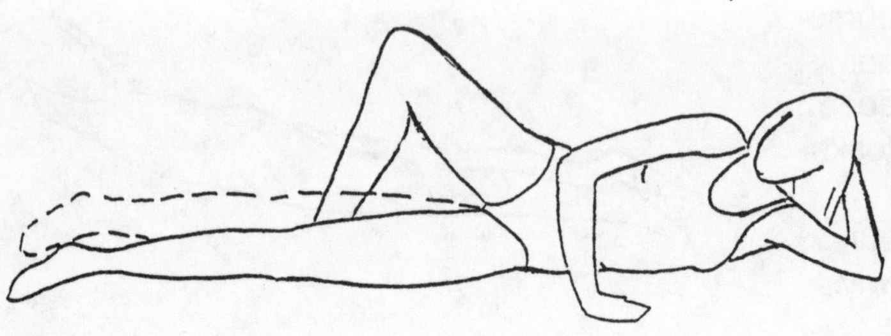

Calf Raises

Keep your knees and hips in a straight line.

Press right up on the ball of your foot.

Stretch your heels down as far as possible.

Return to the stretched position and repeat. Don't bounce.

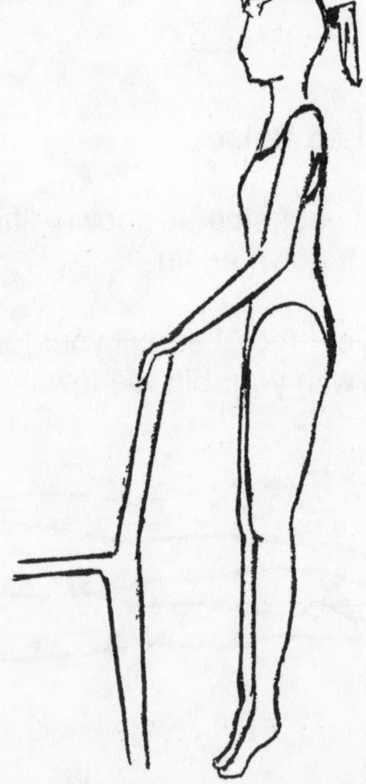

Toe Taps

This exercise is simply pointing and flexing your foot as shown.

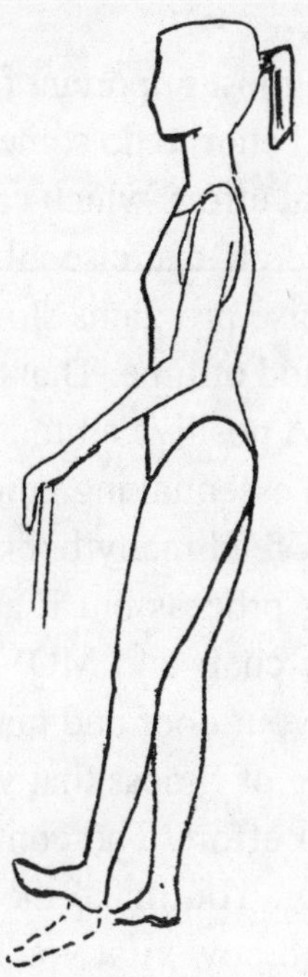

Side Arm Raises

Lift your arms from the side of your body parallel to the floor.

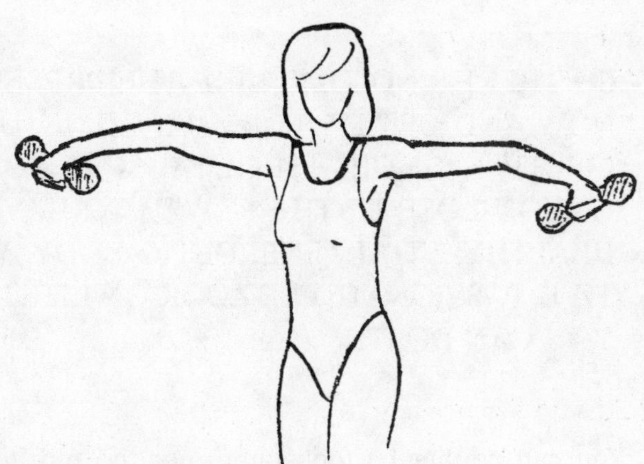

Keep your upper arm in line with your body, fore-arms slightly for-ward and bend your elbows.

Keep your elbows up and turn your thumbs slightly to the door.

Keep your arms in this position, lower them to your sides and repeat.

Added resistance may be used.

One of the most important factors to getting fit is consistency of effort. It is much better to do something every day rather than to kill yourself in one great effort, which can be detrimental and stressful to the body, putting you off exercise all together. (Inch by inch is a cinch). Begin your exercise programs slowly and steadily, increasing your intensity over a period of time. That time will depend on your efforts and determination. A positive attitude is not only necessary in every day activities, it's an essential ingredient of your exercise routine.

You can read many books on fitness, longevity or how to prolong the ageing process but it all comes down to one thing, you have to get off the chair and MOVE! It's up to you! No one will come and knock on your door and make you fit. No pill or potion will give you that feeling of fitness that you'll achieve through discipline, determination and effort. The control to have the body you want is within your power. You make the decision on how you look, how healthy you are and how vital you'll be.

SO THERE'S NO TIME LIKE THE PRESENT! BEGIN IT NOW AND GET FIT FOR A LIFETIME. DON'T TAKE A LIFETIME TO GET FIT BECAUSE IF YOU DON'T USE IT, YOU LOSE IT. THE POWER TO HAVE A STRONG, HEALTHY, VITAL, ENERGETIC BODY, WITH A POSITIVE, PASSIONATE OUTLOOK ON LIFE IS UP TO YOU. YOU CAN DO IT!!

You can neither be too young, nor too old, to improve the efficiency of your body. Regular stretching, strengthening, maintaining ideal posture, keeping aerobically fit and sound nutrition are the keys to good health. As you become fitter you will be surprised how much more energy you have each day to carry out your daily chores. Once you are fully involved in your fitness program you will wonder how you ever lived without it. (Francine St George, *The Muscle Fitness Book).*

This chapter is intended as a guide only and was written by exercise and fitness consultant Ann Mader in collaboration with Dr Sandra Cabot. Before beginning any strenuous physical exercise it is best to seek the advice of your medical practitioner.

References and Suggested Reading:

Balaskis, Arthur & Stirk, John, *Soft Exercise. The Complete Book of Stretching*. Unwin Paperbacks, 1983.

Creager, Joan G., *Human Anatomy and Physiology*. Wadsworth, 1983.

Fitness Health and Nutrition. Time Life Books, 1987.

Fonda, Jane, *Women—Coming of Age*. Viking, 1984.

St George, Francine, *The Muscle Fitness Book*. Simon & Schuster, 1989.

The Body Book, Reader's Digest, 1986.

CHAPTER ELEVEN

DR SANDRA CABOT'S FINE-TUNING 'COCKTAIL'

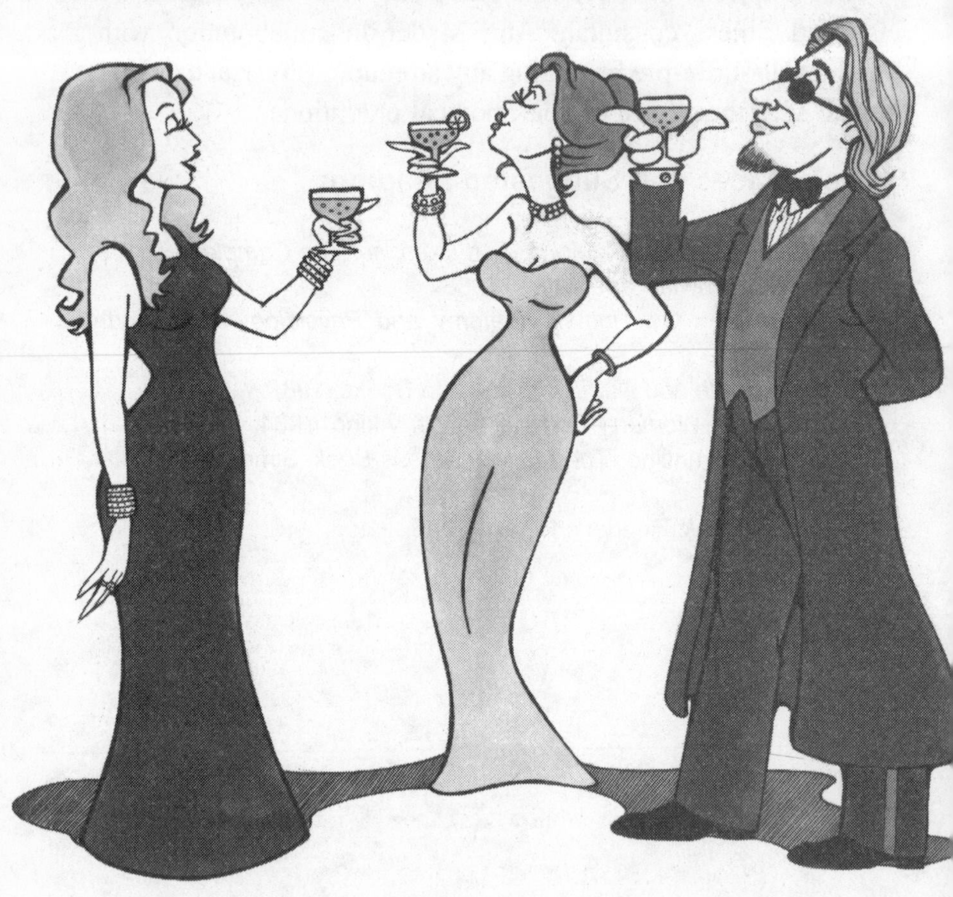

The fine-tuning 'energy cocktail', the new party drink.

I have been in medical practice for well over twenty years and in this time I have used nutritional supplements and dietary modifications to treat my patients far more than prescription drugs. Even if I see a need to prescribe drugs I will always use nutritional medicine as an adjunct to drugs. I have been doing this for a long time, indeed long before it ever became trendy. Many of the patients who have consulted me have been chronically ill and have tried just about everything. In other words they have given me real challenges and have put me 'on the spot' causing me to put on my thinking cap!

I have often been called the 'last resort' or the 'last hope'. Sometimes I have thought it would be easier if they had come just for a sore throat, sickness certificate or a pap smear! These patients have had high expectations and often viewed me as someone with almost magical healing abilities. I sincerely wish that I had these but, unfortunately, I do not. I am not a guru nor am I on a higher level than my medical colleagues who are also faced with great challenges.

However, I am very fortunate as a doctor because I have a long background in nutritional medicine which has given me a wealth of experience and a great faith in natural healing methods. I can usually work out what a patient needs to do to regain their health very quickly as I meet and talk to literally thousands of people through my health seminars and they all relate their histories to me. What is time consuming is convincing them that such simple things as a 'liver-cleansing diet' or an 'energy diet' will have a profoundly positive healing effect.

The most important thing with nutritional medicine is to use its benefits before it is too late. In the early stages of disease it works much more effectively and swiftly, so if you need help get it straight away.

Even if you do need powerful drugs you can still start using nutritional medicine as the two are complementary.

Over the last decade there has been such an explosion in the number and types of natural therapies and supplements on the shelves that many people find it overwhelming. Some promise to be the elixir of youth and perfect health and it is wise to be wary of these as no one supplement can do everything for your cells.

Nature has some basic laws that are always reproducible. For example, to create a thunderstorm you need moist air that is rising because of low atmospheric pressure and if you add heat you will really get a big one. It is the same for our cells, after all these millenia, they still need the same basic raw materials to create efficient metabolism and no one herb or extract (be it pycnogenol or ginkgo) is going to create an efficient cell.

Over the years I have discovered that many patients are unwell because their cells lack the **vital** raw materials to produce efficient metabolism and hence energy production. With this in mind I have created my **'fine-tuning cocktail'** which will ensure that your cells are getting the vital nutrients they need for efficient metabolism/energy production. I have tried to keep this to the bare essentials or if you like the 'energy essentials'.

SPECIAL PRECAUTIONS:

Generally, nutritional supplements are very safe and free of side effects. However, if you have a chronic medical problem you must be guided by your own doctor or health practitioner before taking supplements as you may have individual needs or be taking drugs that could be influenced by nutritional supplements.

For example, those taking anticoagulant drugs, those with a bleeding disorder or low platelets cannot take anything that may reduce blood clotting time even slightly, so they must avoid supplements of vitamin E and/or C and high doses of essential fatty acid capsules. They must get these nutrients from the diet, which is easy if you follow either the liver-cleansing diet or the energy diet.

Those with epilepsy should also avoid high doses of essential fatty acid supplements and obtain essential fatty acids from the diet (see page 71). Those taking certain drugs for osteoporosis such as Rocaltrol or Biphosphonates should not take calcium supplements without their own doctor's approval.

Pregnant women should not take more than 5000 units of vitamin A daily and, generally, should avoid herbs that have powerful effects unless they check with their own doctor first.

Those with auto-immune diseases or severe allergies should be very careful with the herb echinacea and royal jelly.

DR CABOT'S 'FINE-TUNING COCKTAIL'

1. **Vitamin C**, 500 mg daily.

2. **Vitamin E**, 500 IU daily.

3. **Essential fatty acids** from mixed sources such as evening primrose oil, flaxseed oil, blackcurrant seed oil, borage (star flower) oil, cod liver oil. Try to get 3000–4000 mg daily. Vary the sources of these essential fatty acids. Also, you must get essential fatty acids from your diet (see page 71).

4. A complete **magnesium** formula containing a mixture of different types of magnesium, such as magnesium orotate, aspartate, amino acid chelate and phosphate. By taking three to four tablets daily of such a formula you will get 300–400 mg of elemental magnesium daily in an easily absorbed form.

5. **Selenium** in **organic** form such as designer yeast powders to provide 100–200 mcg daily. These powders also provide a good source of other trace minerals, such as boron, manganese, molybdenum, chromium and iodine, as well as the mitochondrial aid maleic acid (see page 125).

6. **Beta carotene** from **organic** sources only, such as carrot juice (one carrot daily is enough), orange coloured fruits and vegetables, raw vegetable juices and/or spirulina, 1000–2000 mg daily. I do

not recommend tablets/capsules of synthetic beta-carotene as they have been proven to be ineffective.

7. If you are not having dairy products I recommend a complete **calcium** formula containing a mixture of different types of calcium to give around 500 mg of elemental calcium daily.

8. If you are highly stressed or drink excessive alcohol, take a good vitamin B complex tablet, three times weekly. Make sure this contains vitamin B_{12}.

9. If your exercise tolerance is poor and you have muscular weakness take **L-carnitine,** 500 mg twice daily on an empty stomach. This will boost production of energy in the mitochondria (metabolic furnaces) inside your cells.

10. If you need a quick or **instant boost of energy** try a combination of these three herbs:
    guarana, 500 mg
    ginseng, 400 mg
    gingko, 100 mg

    These are available combined together in tablets. Take one or two if you have to perform or work and you feel an energy low coming on.

Make sure that you drink plenty of water, especially if you take supplements.

Take supplements at the beginning of meals, immediately before eating.

CHAPTER TWELVE

STRATEGIC TWO-WEEK ENERGY PLAN

WEEK 1

TO STIMULATE METABOLISM

1. **Exercise program.** Brisk walking for 15–20 minutes daily.

   Abdominal curls (see page 190) to increase abdominal tone and so improve motility of large bowel. Do 5–10 of these each day.

   Lower abdominal tucks (see page 191) to increase flow of venous blood back to the heart. Do 5–10 of these each day.

   Those with chronic fatigue may need to reduce the amount of exercise to only a few minutes at a time. They can do slow gentle walking instead of brisk walking

2. Optional: take one **sauna** during this week to increase elimination of toxins via the skin. If you suffer with low blood pressure, are prone to fainting or have heart or kidney disease, do not have a sauna without your doctor's permission.

3. Drink at least two litres of purified or rain **water,** every day, during the day. Sip it slowly in between meals.

4. Have a **raw juice cocktail** twice daily; good combinations are carrot, celery, beetroot, beetroot greens, dandelion greens, apple, spinach. Dilute with water as desired. You will need around 400 ml per day for a cleansing effect.

5. Have a **therapeutic massage** at least once this week and if you have the time have it twice. This will help the elimination of acidic toxins from the muscles and also help your exercise program

.

6. Follow the **recipes found in week one** (see page 76–83). Do not overeat, taking care to only satisfy your hunger.

7. **Nurture your mind and soul.** Take at least one hour daily to do something you enjoy, such as reading, listening to music, making love, being creative, learning to meditate, playing sport, playing with the children or pets, gardening, getting close to nature, or engaging in a passionate hobby. This will increase the endorphin levels in your brain which will generally relax you.

   Do not feel guilty about taking this extra time for yourself and with a bit of luck, you may make it a regular habit!

   Try to feel the feeling of love inside you. Do you remember how you felt when you were 'in love' with another person? Try to recreate this wonderful feeling and direct it towards yourself as well as others. If you are really out of touch with your feelings and feel dead or lifeless and find this impossible, you may want to think about learning to meditate or having some counselling from a psychotherapist. Getting in touch with your innermost loving feelings has a healing effect. Your greatest healer is yourself.

8. **Take a liver tonic** to stimulate elimination of toxins and fat metabolism. Avoid liver tonics containing alcohol and make sure the one you use contains the liver herbs St Mary's thistle, globe artichoke and dandelion, plus the amino acid taurine. Dosage is one teaspoon stirred into fresh juice just before meals twice daily or two capsules just before meals twice daily. Begin with half this dosage and gradually build up to the full dosage during this first week.

9. **Supplements.** Think about the need to take supplements to fine-tune your system. If you have a perfect diet and you feel well all the time, you probably do not need a lot of supplements, provided you can keep up your healthy lifestyle. The only exception to this is if you are pregnant or breast feeding, when it is highly advisable to take supplements of folic acid, a good multivitamin, calcium, iron and essential fatty acids. Also, if you have a family history of cancer I would recommend a daily supplement of anti-oxidants (vitamins A, C, E, and selenium) to reduce your cancer risk.

   But for those who are tired and don't know why, or those with chronic niggling problems that won't go away, I suggest you start on a program similar to my **'fine-tuning cocktail'** (see page 202) which gives you the **energy essentials.** It is a good idea to start with a small dosage, to judge your response. You can begin with one-third to one-half of the suggested doses in my energy cocktail and continue this reduced dose for this first week.

WEEK 2

RESTORATIVE WEEK

1. **Exercise program.**
   Brisk walking for 30 minutes daily.
   Back extension and triceps extension (see page 193 and 192), 5–10 of each daily.
   Side leg raises, 5–10 daily (see page 193).
   Those with chronic fatigue may reduce the amount of exercise according to their tolerance. Even a very small amount of exercise and movement is better than none at all. Some people with chronic fatigue can only muster enough energy to walk around the house and if that is all you can manage, that is fine. Try to increase it by a few minutes daily.

2. **Spirulina hit** (see page 74) in the morning before breakfast.

3. **Energy shake** for breakfast or lunch (see page 73).

4. Continue with the **therapeutic massage,** at least one this week.

5. **Get extra rest.** Go to bed by 9 p.m. and spend 8–10 hours in bed every night.

6. Follow the **recipes** found in the menu plans for **week two** (see pages 84–93). Do not overeat. Eat just enough to satisfy your hunger. Many people dig their grave with their teeth.

7. Do **deep breathing exercises.** Sit in a quiet place, close your eyes and breath deeply and slowly. Concentrate fully on each breath in and out and if thoughts come to distract you, ignore them. Feel the energy in each breath and let it invigorate you. Do this for at least twenty minutes until you feel relaxed. For breathing exercise, see page 138.

8. **Nurture your mind and soul.** Continue to take an hour each day to do something really enjoyable. This will improve your self-esteem and get you back into the habit of loving yourself. Give yourself positive affirmations and leave no room for doubt in your mind. A good affirmation is 'I love and approve of myself and I trust in the process of life' and there are many others that you may like to invent for inspiration.

   Set your goals and visualise them and each day make another step towards your goal. Never give up in the pursuit of your heart's dream and this will keep your passion alive. Keep on searching with an open mind. Although you may be lucky and find someone to help you, it is only your passion and desire that will ever make it happen. Do not expect someone to hand it to you on a platter, as the fulfilment of the dream takes your inspiration and effort. When you can rekindle your own passion and desire you will shine and attract others to assist you.

9. Continue with the **liver tonic** during this week. If the full dosage is too strong and you experience any digestive upset, continue on a reduced dosage. Generally a liver tonic should be taken for eight weeks in the full dosage of one teaspoon twice daily, or two

capsules twice daily. Thereafter it may be continued in a maintenance dose of one teaspoon daily or two capsules daily.

10. **Supplements.** If you have found the supplements helpful, increase the dosage of the supplements to that recommended in the fine-tuning cocktail (see pages 202). If the supplements are having the desired energy-boosting effect you may continue with them at the same dose for eight weeks. After this time, if you are feeling good, you may continue with a maintenance program which is approximately half the dose recommended in the fine-tuning cocktail. If you have medical problems your supplements will need readjusting at regular intervals, so please see your doctor or naturopath regularly.

11. Continue to drink at least eight glasses of **water** daily. This will keep your kidneys healthy, reduce kidney stones and improve your circulation. Water can be taken in the form of filtered water, distilled water, rain water or herbal teas. The body is 90 per cent water and yet we often fail to replenish the fluids lost everyday. Many people are chronically dehydrated which can cause fatigue, headaches and reduced elimination of toxins.

12. **Think about seeing your doctor**, especially if you have not had a check up for one year or more. This is especially true if you are tired and have come to accept this as the 'normal' you. Fatigue can be due to a thousand different causes, such as a hidden cancer or infection, depressive illness, menopause, nutritional deficiencies, diabetes, thyroid disease, auto-immune disease, atherosclerosis, diseases of the heart, lungs, liver or kidneys. These things require expert diagnosis and treatment. Do not neglect your health. This is especially true for men who often have the macho attitude that they will never get sick.

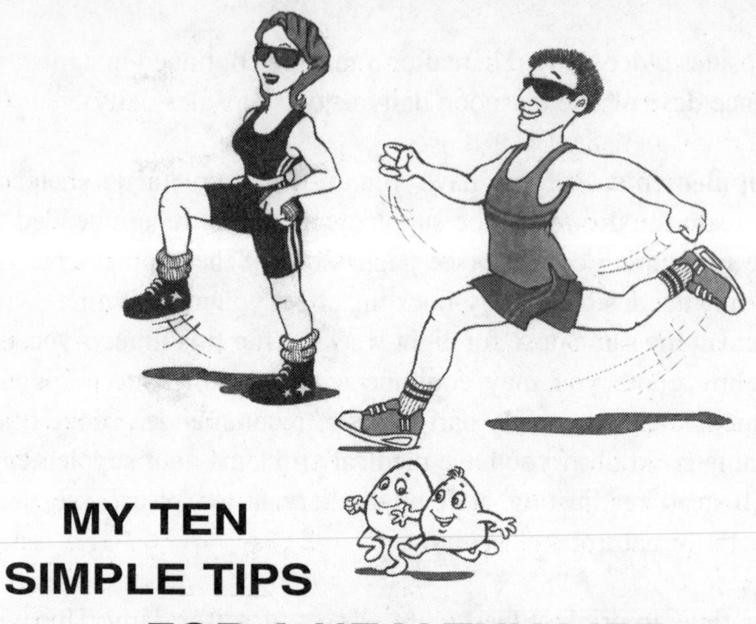

MY TEN SIMPLE TIPS FOR A HEALTHY LIFE

1. Have a thorough annual medical checkup to detect disease in its early and curable stage. You should do this even if you feel extremely well.
2. Always get several expert opinions before committing to major surgery or long-term drug use.
3. Nurture your immune system with a good diet, good hygiene, safe sex and nutritional supplements such as anti-oxidants (vitamin C, E and betacarotene and selenium). A strong immune system is your greatest health asset.
4. Keep up your physical energy with natural food supplements (super foods), such as spirulina, chlorophyll, kelp, garlic, ginseng and nutritional yeast powders and LSA (see page 72). Take supplemental magnesium for its cardiovascular protective properties and to increase energy.
5. Ensure a sufficient intake of good fats, which are essential fatty acids, to increase mental acuity and reduce your chances of dementia in old age. Essential fatty acids are found in beans, legumes, raw nuts, fish, cod liver oil, avocados, lecithin, seeds and their oils (evening primrose oil, starflower oil, flaxseed oil, grapeseed oil, blackcurrant seed oil,

sunflower oil, safflower oil, canola oil.

6. Take regular physical exercise for 30–60 minutes daily. If you have joint pain, swimming and yoga are excellent.
7. Keep a positive state of mind and no matter how difficult problems may seem, try to trust in the process of life and love and approve of yourself. Don't live with depression as modern-day medicine has effective treatments for this common malady.
8. Use the benefits of nutritional medicine to prevent and treat health problems. Over twenty-five years I have seen many chronic and severe diseases overcome with a change in diet and specific nutritional supplements. Seek out a physician who is sympathetic to, or even better, conversant with nutritional medicine. If you become ill, begin using nutritional medicine immediately, as chances of success are much higher.
9. Be aware that in this day and age you do not have to suffer many of the degenerative diseases that we previously considered a normal part of the ageing process. Seek the best advice while you are still healthy. The techniques of hormonal restoration using natural super hormones can slow the ageing process and maintain sexual function.
10. Develop what I call 'liver consciousness' and become aware that you have a liver and take care of it. It is the hardest working organ in your body and a healthy liver will take the load off your immune system and keep your bloodstream clean and your arteries healthy. An efficient liver will also keep your weight under control.

My motto for health is 'love your liver and live longer'.

FAREWELL NOTE

For me, it is a privilege to write for you and of course an even greater privilege if you read my book. Writing is an intimate medium which is a unique way to touch peoples minds and hearts. I do hope that you have enjoyed this book and found inspiration in its pages.

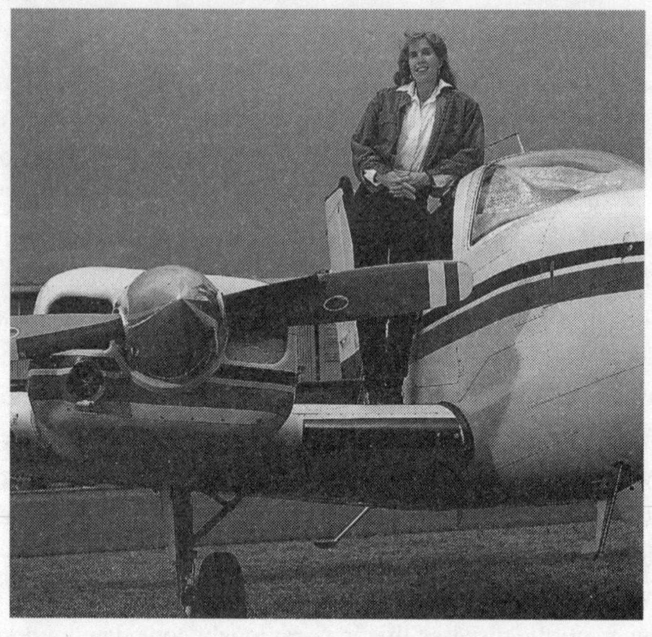

I wish you good health and abundant energy.

I hope to meet you one day in your city.

Sandra Cabot

From the flying doctor.

Yours sincerely,

REFERENCES

1. *Taurine: Orthoplex Research Bulletin*, 'Taurine the Detoxifying Amino Acid', Nutrients in Profile, Henry Osieki, Bioconcepts Publishing.
2. *Australian Journal of Medical Herbalism*, Vol 4 (1), 1992, St Mary's Thistle.
3. *Nutrition Almanac*, fourth edition, McGraw-Hill.
4. *Prescription for Nutritional Healing*, James Balch, Avery Publishing.
5. *Journal of Steroid Biochemistry*, 1986; 25:791–7.
6. *American Journal of Clinical Nutrition*, 1984; 40; 569–78.
   Lancet, 1992; 339; 1233.
7. *The Composition of Foods*, 5th edition, McCance and Widdowson's
   NHAA Newsletter (MEDPLANT abstracts), July 1988.
8. Adlercreutz, H., et al., *Steroid Biochem Molec Biol*. 44, 147, 1993.
   Hansel, R., and Haas, H., Therapie mit phyto-pharmaka, Springer-Verlag, Berlin, 1984.
9. 'Magnesium, The Forgotten Element', Dr Philip Stowell, 5th Oceania Symposium of Complementary Medicine.
10. Buchwald D. and Garrity D., 'Comparison of patients with chronic fatigue syndrome, fibromyalgia and multiple chemical sensitivities', *Arch Intern Med*, 1994; 154:2049–2053.
11. Bland, J.S., Bralley, J.A., 'Nutritional upregulation of hepatic detoxification enzymes', *The Journal of Applied Nutrition*, 1992, 44; No. 3 & 4.
12. Kanazawa, K.,. 'Hepatotoxicity caused by dietary secondary products originating from lipid peroxidation'. In Friedman M., (ed.) *Nutritional and Toxicological Consequences of Food Processing*. New York, NY: Plenum Press; 1991, 237–253.
13. 'Dietary selenium: time to act', *British Medical Journal*, Vol 314, 8/2/1997.
14. 'Effects of Selenium Supplementation for Cancer Prevention in Patients with carcinoma of the skin', *JAMA*, December 25 1996, Vol 276, No. 24.
15. University of California at Berkeley Wellness Letter, Vol 12, Issue 4, January 1996.
16. *Journal of Clinical Endocrinology and Metabolism*, 1990:71, 696–704
17. *Journal of Clinical Obstetrics and Gynaecology* 1977:20, 113–12

18. M.S.George, *Biological Psychiatry*, 1994:35:775–780

19. *Psychoneuro-endocrinology*, Volume 17, No 4, pages 327–333, 1992.

20. G.E. Abraham et.al. *Journal of Nutritional Medicine*, 1992; 3:49–59.

21. James F. Balch, *Prescription for Nutritional Healing*.

22. Stephen Cooter PhD, *Beating Chronic Illness*; Jean Carper, *The Food Pharmacy*;

23. Earl Mindell, *Vitamin Bible*; Walter Schmitt Jr, 'D.C. Molybdenum for candida albicans patients and other problems', *Digest of Chiropractic Economics* 31:4, Jan–Feb, 1991.

24. Boyle E. Jr. et. al, *South Medical Journal*, 1977 Dec; 70 (12):1449–53 ;

25. Mirsky et .al., *Journal Inorg Biochem,* 1980 Aug:13 (1):11–21.

26. Roeback et. al., *Ann Intern Med* 1991 Dec 15:115 (12): 917–24.

27. *Nature Med*, 1995; 1:433–6.

28. Margaret Rayman, *British Medical Journa*l, Vol. 314, 387, Feb,1997.

29 *JAMA*, Vol 276, No. 24, December 1996,

30 *The Physicians Handbook of Clinical Nutrition*, Henry Osiecki, Bioconcepts Publishing.Dec. 1996, Vol 276, No 24.

31. Saiki I, Tohushuma Y, Nishimura K et al, 'Macrophage activation with ubiquinone and their related compounds in mice', *Int. J. Ivit Nutr. Res.* (1983) 53: 312.

32. Folhers K, Morita M, et al, 'The activities of Coenzyme Q10 for immune response', *Biochem. Biophys. Res. Commun*. (1993) May 28, 193 (1) 88–92.

33. Mayer P, Hemberger H, Drews J., 'Differential effect of ubiquinone Q10 on macrophage activation and experimental infections in granulocytopenic mice'. *Infection* (1980) 8:256.

34. Folkers K, et al, 'Increase in levels of IgG in serum of patients treated with Coenzyme Q10', *Res. Comm. Chem. Pathol. Pharmacol* (1982) 38:335.

35. *New England Journal of Medicine*, 1997; 336: 1216–22

36. Allegro et al., *Clinical Trials Journal*, 1987, 24, page 104–108, Oral Phosphatidyl-Serine in elderly subjects with cognitive dysfunction.

37. Crook et al, *Psychopharmacol Bulletin*, 1992, Vol 28, page 61–66, Phosphatidyl-Serine in Alzheimers Disease.

SOME COMMON QUESTIONS and ANSWERS regarding the natural hormones used in troches and creams

Question: Where do the 'natural hormones' used in troches and creams come from and, if they are made in a laboratory how can they be truly natural?

Answer: The 'natural' progesterone, oestrogen and testosterone used in troches and creams are derived from plant hormones (phytosterols). The most common plant hormone used is called diosgenin derived from wild yam and soy beans. This diosgenin is then converted in the laboratory into human hormones, such as progesterone and oestrogen. These hormones are chemically or structurally identical to the sex hormones produced by the human ovary and adrenal gland, so that the body cannot tell the difference. Human ovaries act like hormone laboratories in that they synthesise natural sex hormones. Medical laboratories that synthesise natural hormones in test tubes can be compared to the ovarian and adrenal laboratories in our bodies that synthesise natural hormones, as the end products are identical.

Question: How are 'synthetic' hormones different from 'natural' hormones?

Answer: Synthetic progesterones are called progestogens or progestins and are often derived initially from natural progesterone or testosterone, but they are then further altered in the laboratory by introducing new molecules. This new chemical is more resistant to being broken down by the liver so that it is more potent and longer acting than truly natural hormones. Some women will get side effects from synthetic progestogens, such as depression, weight gain, fluid retention and headaches. Examples of synthetic progestogens are Provera and Primolut. Another progestogen called Duphaston more closely resembles natural progesterone and is less likely to cause side effects. Unfortunately, Duphaston is more expensive than the other synthetic progestogens.

Question: Are the natural hormones used in troches and creams safe?

Answer: There have been no reports of significant side effects or health problems from natural progesterone. Natural oestrogen, pregnenolone and testosterone are hormones and must be prescribed and monitored by a medical doctor, no matter what form they are prescribed in. Thus you must obtain a prescription for natural hormone creams or troches. Any hormones, whether natural or synthetic, can cause side effects if doses are too high or not monitored regularly. For example, natural or synthetic oestrogen in excessive doses can cause fluid retention, heavy bleeding, breast swelling and tenderness and headaches. Natural or synthetic testosterone in excessive doses can cause acne, greasy skin, facial hair, scalp hair loss, deepening of the voice, excessive libido and weight gain. Thus, doses of all types of hormones need to be controlled carefully because they have powerful effects in the body. Generally speaking natural hormones given in the form of troches, tablets, patches or creams are far less likely to cause side effects because smaller doses can be used to fine-tune the individual's hormonal system. Furthermore, natural hormones are more easily broken down by the liver and so do not accumulate in the body and are less potent. Natural progesterone was first manufactured in a laboratory by scientists in the 1930s. Natural oestrogens and testosterone have been used by doctors, particularly in Europe, for over 50 years so they are not new. It is only the way in which we are now able to give these hormones that is new. Remember, you should never treat yourself with hormones, even if they are 'natural', so seek out a doctor well versed in these techniques. For more information call the Hormonal Advisory Service on (02) 4653 1445 or (02) 9387 8111.

Question: Should I have blood tests to see what my hormone levels are?

Answer: Blood tests can be helpful if you are not sure if you are menopausal and this is a common dilemma in women who have had a hysterectomy. If you are currently taking hormone replacement therapy and feel out of balance, or are getting side effects, blood tests are also useful.

The most important tests to have are:

FSH (follicle stimulating hormone)—if levels are above 30 U/L, you are menopausal

Oestradiol (oestrogen)—if levels are consistently less than 50 pmol/L in conjunction with high FSH levels, you are menopausal

FAI (free androgen index)—the normal range is 1–5%. If it is towards the low side, say around 2 or less, you may find benefit from testosterone, especially if you feel very tired and have lost all your libido. DHEA is also of benefit but, unfortunately, is unavailable in Australia.

Question: How do you use natural progesterone to treat premenstrual syndrome?

Answer: It can be administered as a cream containing 4% proges-

terone or as a troche (lozenge) containing 25–100 mg of progesterone.
Dosage: Start treatment on day 14 of your menstrual cycle using ⅛ teaspoon of cream until day 17. From day 18 to 22 use ¼ teaspoon and after this use ½ teaspoon daily until menstrual bleeding begins when you stop using the cream. With 100 mg troches use ¼, ½ and 1 of the troches, in the same sequence. Your own doctor may see fit to use more or less than this, depending upon your symptoms.

Question: What will I do if I get side effects from hormone replacement therapy?

Answer: Side effects such as nausea, weight gain, bloating, fluid retention and headaches are generally a sign that your liver is being overloaded by the extra workload of breaking down the hormones. You may need to reduce the dose or change the proportions of hormones in the troches and you can discuss this with your doctor. Side effects are generally less if creams are used in very sensitive women. Creams can be made containing different hormones all in one cream, such as oestrogen, progesterone and testosterone, for application to the skin or vagina. With creams it is best to massage it into the thinner, softer skin, such as on the inner thighs and upper arms, lower abdomen and neck. Different sites can be rotated to maximise absorption. If you keep getting side effects it is usually a sign that your liver is dysfunctional and needs help. If so, I recommend that you follow my Liver-Cleansing Diet found in one of my books and take a good liver tonic powder containing the herbs St Mary's thistle, globe artichoke and dandelion along with the amino acid taurine. For more information on natural therapies for the liver, call (02) 4653 1445 in Australia or (09) 478 5921 in New Zealand.

Question: What are commonly used dosage protocols for natural hormones?

Answer:	Provera 5 mg	= 100–200 mg natural progesterone
	Provera 10 mg	= 200–400 mg natural progesterone

Starting dose is generally 200 mg daily for menopause or severe premenstrual syndrome.

The natural hormone preparation called Triest is a combination of the three different natural oestrogens produced by the ovaries.

Triest	=	Estriol 80% Estradiol 10% Estrone 10%

Estradiol 1 mg	=	0.3 mg Premarin
Estradiol 2 mg	=	0.625 mg Premarin

EQUIVALENT DOSES

Premarin	Estriol	Tri-estrogen	
0.3 mg	2.5 mg	1.25 mg	
0.625 mg	***5.0 mg***	***2.5 mg***	***Most common dosage***
1.25 mg	7.5 mg	5.0 mg	

AVERAGE HORMONE LEVELS PRESCRIBED BY DOCTORS

Estradiol	1 mg–2 mg	
Triest	1 mg–2 mg	
Testosterone	2 mg–10 mg	***average 5 mg***

U.S.A. READERS -

For information regarding this or other of Dr. Sandra Cabot's books please contact-

SCB INTERNATIONAL
13910 N. FRANK LLOYD WRIGHT BLVD.
SUITE 2A-101
SCOTTSDALE ARIZONA 85260

TOLL FREE NUMBER: 1-888-75 LIVER
e-mail WHANtwrk@aol.com-or see web site - www.whas.com.au- use USA page to order

Information regarding -

FEMMEPHASE Phytoestrogen powder & capsules - (contains natural plant hormones vitamins & minerals.)
LIVATONE - liver tonic - powder & capsules,
SELENOMUNE - designer yeast powder - can also be provided at the above address and phone number.

Network memberships are welcome - (see page 219) at $75 -Australian, payable by Bankcard, MasterCard or Visa

MENOPAUSE

HRT AND ITS NATURAL ALTERNATIVES BY DR SANDRA CABOT

If you would like to send/receive copies of this book to a friend or relative simply fill in this coupon and return it to the WHAS with your payment. The WHAS will then either post it to you or direct to the person you specify on the coupn below. You may cut off the coupon or photocopy it and post it to WHAS.

- -

MAIL THIS COUPON TO: WHAS
155 EAGLE CREEK ROAD, WEROMBI, NSW, AUSTRALIA, 2570

Please send______copies ***Menopause*** at Aust $20 each plus Aust $6.00 for postage and handling.
Please charge my credit card (tick correct card):

☐ BANKCARD ☐ MASTERCARD ☐ VISA

YOUR CREDIT CARD NO:

Card expiry date____________
or find enclosed my cheque/money order payable to WHAS for Aust $__________

Your signature______________________________________

Your name____

Your address____

________________Postcode__________Your telephone no.________________

OR ORDER BY FAX OR TELEPHONE

Telephone: 61 2 4653 1445 or 61 2 4653 1263 to place a credit card order—Bankcard, Mastercard or Visa only accepted.

Fax: 61 2 4653 1144 — fax this completed coupon with your credit card number and personal details filled in.

PERSON YOU WISH *MENOPAUSE* SENT TO:

To whom (name)______________________________________

Address____

____Postcode________________

Please fill in all parts of this coupon, including post codes, and check your credit card number and expiry date before signing. Prompt delivery in a padded bag is assured.

THE BODY-SHAPING DIET

Do you diet and lose weight in the wrong places?
Do you wish to improve your body shape?
Is your cellulite out of control?
Are you getting fat but don't know why?
Are you looking for an easy, safe, economical and nutritious diet?

If so, *The Body-Shaping Diet* is for you!

There are four different body types—ANDROID, GYNAEOID, LYMPHATIC and THYROID—each has distinct hormonal and metabolic differences. To lose weight efficiently and get back your body shape you must follow a diet that has correct food combinations to match YOUR body type. This is called The Body-Shaping Diet.

To order ***The Body-Shaping Diet*** mail this coupon to:

WHAS
155 EAGLE CREEK ROAD, WEROMBI, NSW, AUSTRALIA, 2570
AUSTRALIA

Or order by PHONE 61 2 4653 1445 OR 61 2 4653 1263 or FAX 61 2 4653 1144 using this completed coupon. You need a valid credit card to order by phone or fax.

Please rush me_________copies of ***The Body-Shaping Diet book*** at Aust $20 each plus Aust $6.00 for postage and handling.

Please charge my credit card (tick correct card):

☐ BANKCARD ☐ MASTERCARD ☐ VISA

YOUR CREDIT CARD NO:

Card Expiry Date:__________________

OR find enclosed my cheque/money order payable to WHAS for Aust $______________

Your name:____

Your address____

Postcode____________Your signature____

Only Bankcard, Mastercard or Visa is accepted. Please fill in all parts of this coupon, including post code, credit card number and expiry date before signing.

WOMEN'S HEALTH NETWORK APPLICATION FORM

Do you want to stay in touch with the latest advances in menopause, hormone replacement therapy, anti-ageing techniques, breast care, skin care, nutrition, naturopathic medicine, hormonal problems, improving your sex drive, candida, weight control. body shaping, where to find the best medical specialists and other health issues of vital concern to women?

You can do this by joining our network. This will keep you in touch and give you access to all these things! How?

Through our newsletter and our telephone hot line—61 2 4653 1445 or 61 4 1225 0054

Our friendly, knowledgeable and professional staff will be happy to answer your questions. It really helps when you are talking to someone who understands your dilemmas and can point you in the right direction.

Being a health network member puts you in touch with a network of 'switched on' inspirational and helpful health care workers.

How to join our network!
You can join our Network for 12 months and have all these benefits for only Aust $55.00!

If you want to join, CALL 61 2 4653 1445 or 61 2 4653 1263 or Fax: 61 2 4653 1144 or write to 155 Eagle Creek Road, Werombi, NSW, Australia, 2570

Yes, I want to be a member of The Women's Health Network!

Your Name____

Your Address______________________________________

________________________________Postcode__________

Please charge Aust $55.00 to my credit card (tick correct card)

☐ BANKCARD ☐ MASTERCARD ☐ VISA

YOUR CREDIT CARD NO.: ☐☐☐☐☐☐☐☐☐☐☐☐☐☐☐☐

Card Expiry Date__________

Your phone number__________________________

Your signature______________________________

OR Find enclosed my cheque/money order for Aust $55.00 payable to WHAS

If you would like to discuss liver tonics with a naturopath call

09 478 5921

Or fax your request to

09 478 5991

or write to

PO Box 33–889 Takapuna

An invitation to HAPPINESS in everyday life

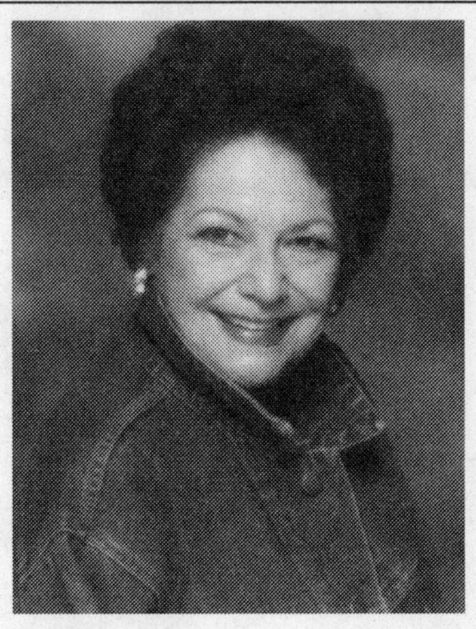

HOW IT WORKS FOR YOU!

Learn to

• Find love! • Keep love!
•& let go! (without feeling sad)

This Little Book Contains Invaluable Knowledge and Practical Strategies for People under Stress & Emotional Strain. It is a Catalyst for the Journey to Self Awareness and Emotional Well being.

—**Dr Sandra Cabot** M.B.B.S. D.R.C.O.G.

Stress In her book Florence says:

"The bottom line is…You have to learn to love yourself! This is the path to Happiness."

An invitation to Happiness in Everyday Life sets out how to reduce your stress levels.

• Work related stress • Relationship stress
• Stress, related to life events

Do you wish to enter an "emotional candy store"?
Florence's book invites you inside.

"Do you want to be happy?" asks Florence. My book shows you how to love and approve of yourself. A recipe for self-confidence.

HOW TO ORDER

An Invitation to Happiness in Everyday Life **by Florence Thomas**
If you require copies of this book or further information write to:
Florence Thomas POBox 990 Randwick Post Office, Randwick, NSW, Australia, 2034

Please feel free to contact me anytime. You can ring me on (02) 9665 1627. I look forward to your call

232